GERIATRICS, GERONTOLOGY AND ELDERLY ISSUES

OLDER PATIENT-DOCTOR COMMUNICATION

GUIDANCE, STRATEGY, TIPS

GERIATRICS, GERONTOLOGY AND ELDERLY ISSUES

Additional books in this series can be found on Nova's website under the Series tab.

Additional e-books in this series can be found on Nova's website under the e-book tab.

GERIATRICS, GERONTOLOGY AND ELDERLY ISSUES

OLDER PATIENT-DOCTOR COMMUNICATION

GUIDANCE, STRATEGY, TIPS

SALLIE H. RYE
EDITOR

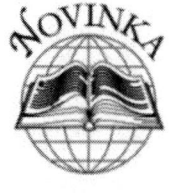

New York

Copyright © 2014 by Nova Science Publishers, Inc.

All rights reserved. No part of this book may be reproduced, stored in a retrieval system or transmitted in any form or by any means: electronic, electrostatic, magnetic, tape, mechanical photocopying, recording or otherwise without the written permission of the Publisher.

For permission to use material from this book please contact us:
Telephone 631-231-7269; Fax 631-231-8175
Web Site: http://www.novapublishers.com

NOTICE TO THE READER

The Publisher has taken reasonable care in the preparation of this book, but makes no expressed or implied warranty of any kind and assumes no responsibility for any errors or omissions. No liability is assumed for incidental or consequential damages in connection with or arising out of information contained in this book. The Publisher shall not be liable for any special, consequential, or exemplary damages resulting, in whole or in part, from the readers' use of, or reliance upon, this material. Any parts of this book based on government reports are so indicated and copyright is claimed for those parts to the extent applicable to compilations of such works.

Independent verification should be sought for any data, advice or recommendations contained in this book. In addition, no responsibility is assumed by the publisher for any injury and/or damage to persons or property arising from any methods, products, instructions, ideas or otherwise contained in this publication.

This publication is designed to provide accurate and authoritative information with regard to the subject matter covered herein. It is sold with the clear understanding that the Publisher is not engaged in rendering legal or any other professional services. If legal or any other expert assistance is required, the services of a competent person should be sought. FROM A DECLARATION OF PARTICIPANTS JOINTLY ADOPTED BY A COMMITTEE OF THE AMERICAN BAR ASSOCIATION AND A COMMITTEE OF PUBLISHERS.

Additional color graphics may be available in the e-book version of this book.

Library of Congress Cataloging-in-Publication Data

ISBN: 978-1-63117-685-2

Published by Nova Science Publishers, Inc. †New York

CONTENTS

Preface   vii

Chapter 1   Talking with Your Older Patient:
A Clinician's Handbook   1
National Institute on Aging

Chapter 2   Talking with Your Doctor:
A Guide for Older People   61
National Institute on Aging

Index   101

PREFACE

Studies find that effective physician-patient communication has specific benefits such as, patients are more likely to adhere to treatment and have better outcomes, they express greater satisfaction with their treatment, and they are less likely to bring malpractice suits. Communicating with older patients involves special issues. The aim of this book is to introduce and/or reinforce communication skills essential in caring for older patients and their families. The book offers practical techniques and approaches to help with diagnosis, promote treatment adherence, make more efficient use of clinicians' time, and increase patient and provider satisfaction. It then continues by discussing ways in which older people should talk to their doctors. A good patient-doctor relationship is more of a partnership. The Book gives a guide on how to ask the right questions to a doctor, along with nurses, physician assistants, pharmacists, and other health care providers, to solve medical problems and keep a patient healthy.

Chapter 1 – Studies find that effective physician-patient communication has specific benefits: patients are more likely to adhere to treatment and have better outcomes, they express greater satisfaction with their treatment, and they are less likely to bring malpractice suits. Research also shows that good communication is a teachable skill. Medical students who receive communication training improve dramatically, not only in communicating with patients, but also in assessing and building relationships with them. Time management skills also get better. Interpersonal and communication skills are now a core competency identified by the Accreditation Council on Graduate Medical Education (ACGME) and the American Board of Medical Specialties (ABMS). Learning effective communication techniques—and using them—

may help you build more satisfying relationships with older patients and become even more skilled at managing their care.

Chapter 2 – In the past, the doctor typically took the lead and the patient followed. Today, a good patient- doctor relationship is more of a partnership. You and your doctor can work as a team, along with nurses, physician assistants, pharmacists, and other health care providers, to solve your medical problems and keep you healthy. This means asking questions if the doctor's explanations or instructions are unclear, bringing up problems even if the doctor doesn't ask, and letting the doctor know if you have concerns about a particular treatment or change in your daily life. Taking an active role in your health care puts the responsibility for good communication on both you and your doctor. All of this is true at any age. But when you're older, it becomes even more important to talk often and comfortably with your doctor. That's partly because you may have more health conditions and treatments to discuss. It's also because your health has a big impact on other parts of your life, and that needs to be talked about too.

Chapter 1

TALKING WITH YOUR OLDER PATIENT: A CLINICIAN'S HANDBOOK*

National Institute on Aging

FOREWORD

Good communication is an important part of the healing process.

Studies find that effective physician-patient communication has specific benefits: patients are more likely to adhere to treatment and have better outcomes, they express greater satisfaction with their treatment, and they are less likely to bring malpractice suits.

Research also shows that good communication is a teachable skill. Medical students who receive communication training improve dramatically, not only in communicating with patients, but also in assessing and building relationships with them. Time management skills also get better. Interpersonal and communication skills are now a core competency identified by the Accreditation Council on Graduate Medical Education (ACGME) and the American Board of Medical Specialties (ABMS).

Learning effective communication techniques—and using them—may help you build more satisfying relationships with older patients and become even more skilled at managing their care.

---

* This is an edited, reformatted and augmented version of NIH Publication No. 08-7105, dated October 2008, reissued September 2011.

Communicating with older patients involves special issues. For example:

- How can you effectively interact with patients facing multiple illnesses and/or hearing and vision impairments?
- What's the best way to approach sensitive topics such as driving privileges or assisted living?
- Are there ways to help older patients who are experiencing confusion or memory loss?

With questions like these in mind, the National Institute on Aging (NIA), part of the National Institutes of Health, developed this booklet.

Although referring to clinicians throughout the text, this booklet is intended for use by a range of professionals dealing directly with patients—physicians, physicians-in-training, nurse practitioners, nurses, physician assistants, and other health care professionals. The aim is to introduce and/or reinforce communication skills essential in caring for older patients and their families. *Talking With Your Older Patient: A Clinician's Handbook* offers practical techniques and approaches to help with diagnosis, promote treatment adherence, make more efficient use of clinicians' time, and increase patient and provider satisfaction.

Three points are important to remember:

- Stereotypes about aging and old age can lead patients and health professionals alike to dismiss or minimize problems as an inevitable part of aging. What we're learning from research is that aging alone does not cause illness and that growing older does not automatically mean having to live with pain and discomfort.
- Many of this booklet's suggestions may, at first glance, appear to be time-consuming, especially given the time constraints of most clinicians. However, an initial investment of time can lead to long-term gains for physicians and patients. Time-intensive practices need not be inefficient. You may get to know your older patient's life history over the course of several visits rather than trying to get it all in one session.
- Older patients are diverse and unique, just like your younger patients. You may see frail 60-year-olds and relatively healthy 80-year-olds. Your patients may be culturally diverse. Some may be quite active while others may be sedentary. The techniques offered here encourage

you to view all older people as individuals who have a wide range of health care needs and questions.

Many physicians, nurses, researchers, and other health care professionals were generous in providing information and advice on making this edition of the *Clinician's Handbook* useful. The Institute is grateful for their thoughtful contributions.

Richard J. Hodes, M.D., Director
National Institute on Aging
National Institutes of Health

CONSIDERING HEALTH CARE PERCEPTIONS

The best way to learn what is and is not acceptable is to communicate directly with patients and caregivers.

> "I'm 30 . . . until I look in the mirror."
>
> Mrs. Hill is an 85-year-old nursing home resident. She has lived in a facility since advanced heart disease made it impossible for her to live independently. Her adult children feel that life in a nursing home must be a nightmare. They want to do something, but they don't know what. Moving her to one of their homes isn't an option; visiting her makes them feel depressed. One day, her doctor chats with Mrs. Hill about life in the home. She tells him that this is one of the best times of her life—people prepare and deliver her meals, she has a comfortable room with a view of the gardens, and the place is very peaceful. Mrs. Hill is quite happy and has no desire to move.

For Mrs. Hill, a life her children find unacceptable is, in fact, just fine with her. What seems intolerable to a 40-year-old may actually be preferred by a 90-year-old.

In the past century, the nature of old age has changed dramatically. In the early 1900s, the average life expectancy was about 49 years—today, it is nearly 80 years. With longevity, however, comes the sobering news that older people may live for years with one or more chronic, potentially disabling conditions. This means they will have an ongoing need for medical services.

No single characteristic describes an older patient. Each person has a different view of what it means to be old. A 68-year-old woman with an active consulting business is likely to deal with a visit to the doctor quite differently from her frail 88-year-old aunt who rarely ventures beyond her neighborhood.

The perspectives that follow are common among older people—and important to consider when talking with older patients.

Views of Physicians and Clinicians

In the past, older people have held doctors in high esteem and treated them with deference. This view may change over time as aging baby boomers are likely to take a more egalitarian and active approach to their own health care.

Today, many older people don't want to "waste the doctor's time" with concerns they think the clinician will deem unimportant. Patients sometimes worry that if they complain too much about minor issues, they won't be taken seriously later on. Or, they are afraid of the diagnosis or treatment. They may worry that the physician will recommend surgery or suggest costly diagnostic tests or medications.

Some patients do not ask questions for fear of seeming to challenge the clinician. On the other hand, some older people, having ample time and interest, will bring popular medical articles to the attention of their providers. This kind of active patient participation can provide an opportunity for communication.

Views of Aging

Ageism can work both ways. Doctors can make assumptions about their older patients. Older people may unwittingly assume the stereotypes of old age. Expectations regarding health diminish with age, sometimes realistically, but often not. Older people with treatable symptoms may dismiss their problems as an inevitable part of aging and not get medical care. As a result, they may suffer needless discomfort and disability. Some may not even seek treatment for serious conditions.

The process of aging may be troubling for older adults. It can be especially hard for people who once bounced back quickly from an illness or were generally healthy. Experts observe that baby boomers bring different expectations, experiences, and preferences to aging than did previous generations. For instance, some boomers are likely to want to participate actively in health care treatments and decisions. They may also search the Internet for health information.

Values about Health

Although physicians typically focus primarily on diagnosing and treating disease, older people generally care most about maintaining the quality of their lives. They are not necessarily preoccupied with death. In fact, many older people are relatively accepting of the prospect of death and seek chiefly to make the most of their remaining years. Younger family members, who commonly must make life-and-death decisions when an older person is incapacitated, may be unaware of the patient's views and preferences.

In Summary

- Let older patients know that you welcome their questions and participation.
- Encourage older adults to voice their concerns.
- Be alert to barriers to communication about symptoms, such as fears about loss of independence or costs of diagnostic tests.
- Expect those in the baby boom generation to be more active participants in their health care.

UNDERSTANDING OLDER PATIENTS

What was once called "bedside manner" and considered a matter of etiquette and personal style has now been the subject of a large number of empirical studies. The results of these studies suggest that the interview is integral to the process and outcomes of medical care.

> **"Tell me more about how you spend your days."**
>
> Although she complains of her loneliness and long days in front of the TV, Mrs. Klein refuses to participate in activities at the community senior center. "I'm not playing bingo with a bunch of old ladies," she tells her doctor when he suggests she get out more. "You've mentioned how much you love to garden," her doctor says. "The center has a garden club with a master gardener. One of my other patients says she loves it." "I don't want to hang around old people who have nothing better to do than compare health problems," she says. "Why not give it a try?" her doctor asks. "You might find the members are pretty active gardeners." Six months later, when she sees the doctor again, Mrs. Klein thanks him. She has joined the garden club and reports that the members all have green thumbs as well as being quite lively conversationalists. Better still, Mrs. Klein's depressive symptoms seem improved.

Effective communication has practical benefits. It can:

- help prevent medical errors
- strengthen the patient-provider relationship
- make the most of limited interaction time
- lead to improved health outcomes

This section provides tips on how to communicate with older patients in ways that are respectful and informative.

Use Proper Form of Address

Establish respect right away by using formal language. As one patient said, *"Don't call me Edna, and I won't call you Sonny."* You might ask your patient about preferred forms of address and how she or he would like to address you. Use Mr., Mrs., Ms., and so on. Avoid using familiar terms, like "dear" and "hon," which tend to sound patronizing. Be sure to talk to your staff about the importance of being respectful to all of your patients, especially those who are older and perhaps used to more formal terms of address.

Make Older Patients Comfortable

Ask staff to make sure patients have a comfortable seat in the waiting room and help with filling out forms if necessary. Be aware that older patients may need to be escorted to and from exam rooms, offices, and the waiting area. Staff should check on them often if they have to wait long in the exam room.

Take a Few Moments to Establish Rapport

Introduce yourself clearly. Show from the start that you accept the patient and want to hear his or her concerns. If you are a consultant in a hospital setting, remember to explain your role or refresh the patient's memory of it.

In the exam room, greet everyone and apologize for any delays. With new patients, try a few comments to promote rapport: *"Are you from this area?"* or *"Do you have family nearby?"* With established patients, friendly questions about their families or activities can relieve stress.

Try Not to Rush

Avoid hurrying older patients. Time spent discussing concerns will allow you to gather important information and may lead to improved cooperation and treatment adherence.

Feeling rushed leads people to believe that they are not being heard or understood. Be aware of the patient's own tendency to minimize complaints or to worry that he or she is taking too much of your time.

Avoid Interrupting

One study found that doctors, on average, interrupt patients within the first 18 seconds of the initial interview. Once interrupted, a patient is less likely to reveal all of his or her concerns. This means finding out what you need to know may require another visit or some follow-up phone calls.

Older people may have trouble following rapid-fire questioning or torrents of information. By speaking more slowly, you will give them time to process what is being asked or said. If you tend to speak quickly, especially if your accent is different from what your patients are used to hearing, try to slow down. This gives them time to take in and better understand what you are saying.

Use Active Listening Skills

Face the patient, maintain eye contact, and when he or she is talking, use frequent, brief responses, such as *"okay," "I see,"* and *"uh-huh."* Active listening keeps the discussion focused and lets patients know you understand their concerns.

Demonstrate Empathy

Watch for opportunities to respond to patients' emotions, using phrases such as *"That sounds difficult"* or *"I'm sorry you're facing this problem; I think we can work on it together."* Studies show that empathy can be learned and practiced and that it adds less than a minute to the patient interview. It also has rewards in terms of patient satisfaction, understanding, and adherence to treatment.

For more information on active listening, contact

American Academy on Communication in Healthcare
16020 Swingley Ridge Road, Suite 300
Chesterfield, MO 63017
1-636-449-5080
www.aachonline.org

This professional organization aims to improve physician-patient relationships and offers courses and publications on medical encounters and interviews.

Macy Initiative in Health Communication
Division of Primary Care
NYU School of Medicine

550 First Avenue
Old Bellevue, Room D401
New York, NY 10016
1-212-263-3071
http://macyinitiative.med.nyu.edu

This initiative was a collaborative effort of three medical schools to identify and define critical communication skills needed by physicians. It developed competency-based curricula for medical students.

New England Research Institutes (NERI)
9 Galen Street
Watertown, MA 02472
1-617-923-7747
www.neriscience.com

NERI has designed a CME-accredited CD-ROM, *Communicating With Older Adults*, educating physicians on communication strategies to practice with older patients.

Avoid Jargon

Try not to assume that patients know medical terminology or a lot about their disease. Introduce necessary information by first asking patients what they know about their condition and building on that. Although some terms seem commonplace—MRIs, CAT scans, stress tests, and so on—some older patients may be unfamiliar with what each test really is. Check often to be sure that your patient understands what you are saying. You may want to spell or write down diagnoses or important terms to remember.

Reduce Barriers to Communication

Older adults often have sensory impairments that can affect communication. Vision and hearing problems need to be treated and accounted for in communication. Ask older patients when they last had vision and hearing exams.

COMPENSATING FOR HEARING DEFICITS

Age-related hearing loss is common. About one-third of people between the ages of 65 and 75, and nearly half of those over the age of 75, have a hearing impairment. Here are a few tips to make it easier to communicate with a person who has lost some hearing:

- Make sure your patient can hear you. Ask if the patient has a working hearing aid. Look at the auditory canal for the presence of excess earwax.
- Talk slowly and clearly in a normal tone. Shouting or speaking in a raised voice actually distorts language sounds and can give the impression of anger.
- Avoid using a high-pitched voice; it is hard to hear.
- Face the person directly, at eye level, so that he or she can lip-read or pick up visual clues.
- Keep your hands away from your face while talking, as this can hinder lip- reading ability.
- Be aware that background noises, such as whirring computers and office equipment, can mask what is being said.
- If your patient has difficulty with letters and numbers, give a context for them. For instance, say, "'m' as in Mary, 'two' as in twins, or 'b' as in boy." Say each number separately (e.g., "five, six" instead of "fifty-six"). Be especially careful with letters that sound alike (e.g., m and n, and b, c, d, e, t, and v).
- Keep a note pad handy so you can write what you are saying. Write out diagnoses and other important terms.
- Tell your patient when you are changing the subject. Give clues such as pausing briefly, speaking a bit more loudly, gesturing toward what will be discussed, gently touching the patient, or asking a question.

COMPENSATING FOR VISUAL DEFICITS

Visual disorders become more common as people age. Here are some things you can do to help manage the difficulties caused by visual deficits:

- Make sure there is adequate lighting, including sufficient light on your face. Try to minimize glare.
- Check that your patient has brought and is wearing eyeglasses, if needed.
- Make sure that handwritten instructions are clear.
- When using printed materials, make sure the type is large enough and the typeface is easy to read. The following print size works well:

"This size is readable."

- If your patient has trouble reading, consider alternatives such as tape recording instructions, providing large pictures or diagrams, or using aids such as specially configured pillboxes.

Be Careful About Language

Some words may have different meanings to older patients than to you or your peers. For example, the word "dementia" may connote insanity, and the word "cancer" may be considered a death sentence. Although you cannot anticipate every generational difference in language use, being aware of the possibility may help you to communicate more clearly. Use simple, common language, and ask if clarification is needed. Offer to repeat or reword the information: *"I know this is complex; I'll do my best to explain, but let me know if you have any questions or just want me to go over it again."*

For more information on low literacy, contact

Partnership for Clear Health Communication
National Patient Safety Foundation
268 Summer Street, 6th Floor
Boston, MA 02210
1-617-391-9900
www.npsf.org/askme3

This national coalition addresses issues related to low health literacy and its effect on outcomes. Its "Ask Me 3" campaign has materials for physicians' offices, including patient handouts, to promote good communication.

Low literacy or inability to read also may be a problem. Reading materials written at an easy reading level may help.

Ensure Understanding

Conclude the visit by making sure the patient understands:

- what the main health issue is
- what he or she needs to do about it
- why it is important to do it

One way to do this is the "teach-back method"—ask patients to say what they understand from the visit. Also, ask if there is anything that might keep the patient from carrying out the treatment plan.

In Summary

- Address the patient by last name, using the title the patient prefers (Mr., Ms., Mrs., etc.).
- Begin the interview with a few friendly questions not directly related to health.
- Don't rush, and try not to interrupt; speak slowly, and give older patients a few extra minutes to talk about their concerns.
- Use active listening skills.
- Avoid jargon, use common language, and ask if clarification is needed, such as writing something down.
- Ask the patient to say what he or she understands about the problem and what needs to be done.

OBTAINING THE MEDICAL HISTORY

When patients are older, obtaining a good history—including information on social circumstances and lifestyle as well as medical and family history—is crucial to sound health care.

> **"What brings you here today?"**
> Mr. Symonds has advanced lung disease and usually manages well with home oxygen. But, he's been admitted to the emergency room three times in as many weeks, unable to breathe. The health team is puzzled because Mr. Symonds is taking his medications on schedule and, he says, using the oxygen. Finally, a home care nurse is sent to the Symonds' house. She discovers that because of this winter's bitter cold, Mr. Symonds has been running a kerosene heater in his kitchen. He does not use the oxygen and heater at the same time for fear of fire.

The varied needs of older patients may require different interviewing techniques. The following guidelines can help you to obtain a thorough history of current and past concerns, family history, medications, and socioeconomic situation. These suggestions are less time-consuming than they may appear. Some involve a single investment of time. Other health care professionals in the office or home may assist in gathering the information. You may want to get a detailed life and medical history as an ongoing part of older patients' office visits and use each visit to add to and update information.

General Suggestions

You may need to be especially flexible when obtaining the medical history of older patients. Here are some strategies to make efficient use of your time and theirs:

- If feasible, try to gather preliminary data before the session. Request previous medical records or, if there is time, mail forms that the patient or a family member can complete at home. Try to structure questionnaires for easy reading by using large type and providing enough space between items for people to respond. Questionnaires to fill out in the waiting room should be brief.
- Try to have the patient tell his or her story only once, not to another staff member and then again to you. For older patients who are ill, this process can be very tiring.
- Sit and face the patient at eye level. Use active listening skills, responding with brief comments such as *"I see"* and *"okay."*
- Be willing to depart from the usual interview structure. You might understand the patient's condition more quickly if you elicit his or her

past medical history immediately after the chief complaint, before making a complete evaluation of the present illness.
- If the patient has trouble with open-ended questions, make greater use of yes-or-no or simple choice questions.
- Remember that the interview itself can be beneficial. Although you see many patients every day, you may be the only person your patient is socially engaged with that day. Your attention is important. Giving your patient a chance to express concerns to an interested person can be therapeutic.

Elicit Current Concerns

Older patients tend to have multiple chronic conditions. They may have vague complaints or atypical presentations. Thinking in terms of current concerns rather than a chief complaint may be helpful. You might start the session by asking your patient to talk about his or her major concern, *"Tell me, what is bothering you the most?"*

Resist the Tendency to Interrupt

Give the patient time to answer your questions. Giving someone uninterrupted time to express concerns enables him or her to be more open and complete.

Probe

Ask, *"Is there anything else?"* This question, which you may have to repeat several times, helps to get all of the patient's concerns on the table at the beginning of the visit.

The main concern may not be the first one mentioned, especially if it is a sensitive subject. If there are too many concerns to address in one visit, you can plan with the patient to address some now and some next time.

Encourage the patient and his or her caregivers to bring a written list of concerns and questions. Sometimes an older patient will seek medical care because of concerns of family members or caregivers.

Ask about Medications

Side effects, interactions, and misuse of medications can lead to major complications in older people. It is crucial to find out which prescription and over-the-counter medications older patients are using and how often. Older people often take many medications prescribed by several different doctors, e.g., internists, cardiologists, urologists, or rheumatologists. Sometimes they take prescriptions intended for other household members.

Remember to ask about any alternative treatments, such as dietary supplements, homeopathic remedies, or teas that the patient might be using. Remind patients that it is important for you to know what over-the-counter medicines, such as pain relievers or eye drops, they use.

Ask patients to bring all medications, both prescription and over-the-counter, to your office. A good approach is to have the patient put everything he or she takes in a brown bag and bring it to each visit. Find out about the patient's habits for taking each medication, and check to be sure that he or she is using it as directed.

Check to see if the patient has (or needs) a medical alert ID bracelet or necklace. There are several sources, including MedicAlert Foundation International, www.medicalert.org.

Obtain a Thorough Family History

The family history is valuable, in part because it gives you an opportunity to explore the patient's experiences, perceptions, and attitudes regarding illness and death. For example, a patient may say, "I never want to be in a nursing home like my mother." Be alert for openings to discuss issues such as advance directives.

The family history not only indicates the patient's likelihood of developing some diseases but also provides information on the health of relatives who care for the patient or who might do so in the future.

Knowing the family structure will help you to know what support may be available from family members, if needed.

Ask about Functional Status

Knowing an older patient's usual level of functioning and learning about any recent significant changes are fundamental to providing appropriate health care. They also influence which treatment regimens are suitable. The ability to perform basic activities of daily living (ADLs) reflects and affects a patient's health. Depending on the patient's status, ask about ADLs such as eating, bathing, and dressing and more complex instrumental activities of daily living (IADLs) such as cooking, shopping, and managing finances. There are standardized ADL assessments that can be done quickly and in the office.

Sudden changes in ADLs or IADLs are valuable diagnostic clues. If your older patient stops eating, becomes confused or incontinent, or stops getting out of bed, look for underlying medical problems. Keep in mind the possibility that the problem may be acute.

Consider a Life History

If you plan to continue caring for an older patient, consider taking time to learn about his or her life. A life history is an excellent investment. It helps to understand the patient. It also strengthens the clinician-patient relationship by showing your interest in the patient as a person.

Be alert for information about the patient's relationships with others, thoughts about family members or coworkers, typical responses to stress, and attitudes toward aging, illness, work, and death. This information may help you interpret the patient's concerns and make appropriate recommendations.

Obtain a Social History

The social history also is crucial. If you are aware of your patient's living arrangements or his/her access to transportation, you are much more likely to devise realistic, appropriate interventions. Ask about where he or she lives; neighborhood safety; eating habits; tobacco, drug, and alcohol use; typical daily activities; and work, education, and financial situations. It also helps to find out who lives with or near the patient.

Understanding a person's life and daily routine can help you to understand how your patient's lifestyle might affect his or her health care. To this end, determine if the patient is an informal caregiver for others. Many older people care for spouses, elderly parents, or grandchildren. A patient's willingness to report symptoms sometimes depends on whether the patient thinks he or she can "afford to get sick," in view of family responsibilities.

House calls by a health care professional are an excellent way to find out about a patient's home life. If that's not possible, try to learn some details about the patient's home life: *"Do you use oil or gas heat? Have steep stairs to navigate? Own a pet? Can you get to the grocery store or pharmacy on your own? Are you friendly with anyone in the neighborhood?"* Learning about your patient's home life will help you understand aspects of his or her illness and may improve adherence to treatment.

In Summary

- Obtain basic information before the visit. Encourage patients to bring in written lists of concerns as well as all medication, including over-the-counter and alternative or homeopathic remedies.
- Use the family history to gain insight into an older patient's social situation as well as his or her risk of disease.
- Talk about the activities of daily living and be alert to changes.
- Ask about living arrangements, transportation, and lifestyle to help in devising appropriate interventions.

ENCOURAGING WELLNESS

People of all ages can benefit from healthy habits such as regular exercise and good nutrition.

> **"I'd like you to try this exercise routine. Just start low and go slow."**
>
> Mrs. Green is surprised when Dr. Lipton recommends that she exercise regularly. She responds with a list of excuses: exercise is for young people, it's not safe for people over 65, it takes too much time, exercise equipment costs too much. Dr. Lipton listens empathetically and then tells her that exercise and physical activity are good for people of all ages and that being sedentary is far more dangerous than exercising.

> He explains that Mrs. Green can "start low and go slow" by walking for 10 minutes at a time and building up to at least 30 minutes of physical activity on 5 days or more each week. At her next office visit, Mrs. Green says that she has more energy than she used to; in fact, she's ready to try a dance class at her senior center.

Exercise and Physical Activity

Exercise has proven benefits for older people. It reduces risk of cardiovascular disease, stroke, hypertension, type 2 diabetes, osteoporosis, obesity, colon cancer, and breast cancer. It also decreases the risk of falls and fall-related injuries.

Like the rest of us, older people may know that exercise is good for their health, but may not have the motivation or encouragement to do it. You can guide your patients by asking about their daily activities and whether they engage in any kind of regular exercise or physical activity.

> ### TOO OLD TO EXERCISE? STUDIES SAY 'NO!'
>
> - Together, exercise and lifestyle changes such as becoming more active and healthy eating reduce the risk of diabetes in high-risk older people. In one study, lifestyle changes led to a 71 percent decrease in diabetes among people 60 and older.
> - In another study, moderate exercise was effective at reducing stress and sleep problems in older women caring for a family member with dementia.
> - Older people who exercise moderately are able to fall asleep quickly, sleep for longer periods, and get better quality of sleep.
> - Researchers also found that exercise, which can improve balance, reduced falls among older people by 33 percent.
> - Walking and strength-building exercises by people with knee osteoarthritis help reduce pain and maintain function and quality of life.

There are several ways to encourage older patients to exercise:

- Whenever appropriate, let them know that regular physical activity—including endurance, muscle-strengthening, balance, and flexibility exercises—is essential for healthy aging.
- Help patients set realistic goals and develop an exercise plan.
- Write an exercise prescription, and make it specific, including type, frequency, intensity, and time; follow up to check progress and re-evaluate goals over time.
- Refer patients to community resources, such as mall-walking groups and senior center fitness classes.

Tell them about *Go4Life^{TM}*, NIA's exercise and physical activity campaign. It has exercises, motivational tips, and free materials to help older adults start exercising and keep going. Check out www.nia.nih.gov/Go4Life.

For more information on exercise, nutrition, and older people, contact

Centers for Disease Control and Prevention (CDC)
1600 Clifton Road
Atlanta, Georgia 30333
1-800-232-4636 (toll-free)
1-888-232-6348 (TTY/toll-free) Healthy Aging: www.cdc.gov/aging
Nutrition, Physical Activity, and Obesity: www.cdc.gov/nccdphp/dnpao

The CDC has resources on nutrition and physical activity for older adults. The Division of Nutrition, Physical Activity, and Obesity addresses how healthy eating habits and exercise can improve the public's health and prevent and control chronic diseases.

Department of Agriculture
Food and Nutrition Information Center (FNIC)
National Agricultural Library
10301 Baltimore Avenue, Room 105
Beltsville, MD 20705
1-301-504-5414
www.nal.usda.gov/fnic

The FNIC website provides over 2,000 links to current and reliable nutrition resources.

**National Institute on Aging (NIA)
Information Center**
P.O. Box 8057
Gaithersburg, MD 20898-8057
1-800-222-2225 (toll-free)
1-800-222-4225 (TTY/toll-free)
www.nia.nih.gov/health www.nia.nih.gov/Go4Life

NIA has free online and print materials to show older adults how to start and maintain a safe, effective program of endurance, flexibility, balance, and strength-training exercises.

National Resource Center on Nutrition, Physical Activity & Aging
Florida International University
OE 200
Miami, FL 33199
1-305-348-1517
http://nutritionandaging.fiu.edu

A group serving nutrition programs funded by the Older Americans Act, the Center aims to increase food and nutrition services in home- and community-based social, health, and long- term-care systems serving older adults. Link to the program "Eat Better & Move More."

Nutrition

Older patients may develop poor eating habits for many reasons. These can range from a decreased sense of smell and taste to teeth problems or depression. Older people may also have difficulty getting to a supermarket or standing long enough to cook a meal. And although energy needs may decrease with age, the need for certain vitamins and minerals, including calcium, vitamin D, and vitamins B_6 and B_{12}, increases after age 50.

Try these strategies to encourage healthy diets:

- Emphasize that good nutrition can have an impact on well-being and independence.
- If needed, suggest liquid nutrition supplements, but emphasize the benefits of solid foods.

- If needed, suggest multivitamins that fulfill 100 percent of the recommended daily amounts of vitamins and minerals for older people, but not megadoses.
- Offer a referral to a nutrition services program, such as Meals on Wheels. Programs in your area are provided by the local Area Agency on Aging or Tribal Senior Services. Contact Eldercare Locator at 1-800-677-1116 for your Area Agency on Aging.

In Summary

- Talk to your older patients about the importance of exercise and physical activity. Staying active can benefit older people in many ways.
- Encourage your patients to get a free copy of *Exercise and Physical Activity: Your Everyday Guide from the National Institute on Aging*.
- Talk to your older patients about their eating habits.
- Consider having your older patients keep a food diary, if necessary, to make sure they are getting the correct nutrients.

TALKING ABOUT SENSITIVE SUBJECTS

Caring for an older patient requires discussing sensitive topics. You may be tempted to avoid these discussions, but there are helpful techniques to get you started and resources to help.

"Many people your age experience similar problems."

At age 80, Mr. Abayo was proud of his independence and ability to get around. But, when he came to see Dr. Carli for a regular exam, he acknowledged that the trouble with his shoulder had started after he collided with another car at a four-way stop sign. "Many of my patients are worried about being safe drivers," Dr. Carli said. After the exam, she spoke with Mr. Abayo and his son in her office.

> She told them that a lot of her older patients had decided to rely on family and friends for transportation. She gave Mr. Abayo a pamphlet on older drivers and the number of a local transportation resource that might be helpful.

Many older people have a "don't ask, don't tell" relationship with health care providers about some problems, especially those related to sensitive subjects, such as driving, urinary incontinence, or sexuality. Hidden health issues, such as memory loss or depression, are a challenge. Addressing problems related to safety and independence, such as giving up one's driver's license or moving to assisted living, also can be difficult.

You may feel awkward addressing some of these concerns because you don't know how to help patients solve the problem. This section gives an overview of techniques for broaching sensitive subjects, as well as resources for more information or support.

Try to take a universal, non-threatening approach. Start by saying, *"Many people your age experience . . ."* or *"Some people taking this medication have trouble with . . ."* Try: *"I have to ask you a lot of questions, some that might seem silly. Please don't be offended . . ."* Another approach is to tell anecdotes about patients in similar circumstances as a way to ease your patient into the discussion, of course always maintaining patient confidentiality to reassure the patient you are talking to that you won't disclose personal information about him or her.

Some patients avoid issues that they think are inappropriate for their own clinicians. One way to overcome this is to keep informative brochures and materials readily available in the waiting room. Along with each topic listed alphabetically below is a sampling of resources. Although the lists are not exhaustive, they are a starting point for locating useful information and referrals.

Advance Directives

Advance directives, including "living wills," can help you honor individual end-of-life preferences and desires. You may feel uncomfortable raising the issue, fearing that patients will assume the end is near. But, in fact, this is a conversation that is best begun well before end-of-life care is appropriate. Let your patients know that advance care planning is a part of good health care. You can say that, increasingly, people realize the importance of making plans while they are still healthy. You can let them know that these plans can be revised and updated over time or as their health changes.

An advance care planning discussion can take about 5 minutes with a healthy patient:

- Talk about the steps your patient would want you to take in the event of certain conditions or eventualities.
- Discuss the meaning of a health care proxy and how to select one.
- Give the patient the materials to review, complete, and return at the next visit. In some cases, the patient may want help completing the form.
- Ask the patient to bring a copy of the completed form at the next visit for you to keep. If appropriate, share the plan with family members.
- Revise any advance directives based on the patient's changing health and preferences.

Be sure to put a copy of the completed form in the medical record. Too often, forms are completed, but when needed, they cannot be found. Many organizations now photocopy the forms on neon-colored paper, which is easy to spot in the medical record.

If your patient is in the early stages of an illness, it's important for you to assess whether or not the underlying process is reversible. It's also a good time to discuss how the illness is likely to play out. If your patient is in the early stages of a cognitive problem, it is especially important to discuss advance directives.

For more information on advance directives, contact

Aging with Dignity
P.O. Box 1661
Tallahassee, FL 32302-1661
1-888-594-7437 (toll-free)
www.agingwithdignity.org
This group provides an easy-to-read advance care planning document called Five Wishes.

Institute for Healthcare Advancement
501 South Idaho Street, Suite 300
La Habra, CA 90631

1-800-434-4633 (toll-free)
www.iha4health.org
A simplified advance directive form written at a fifth-grade reading level in English, Spanish, Chinese, and Vietnamese can be downloaded for free.

National Hospice and Palliative Care Organization
1731 King Street, Suite 100
Alexandria, VA 22314
1-800-658-8898 (toll-free)
1-877-658-8896 (toll-free, multilingual helpline)
www.caringinfo.org
This group provides resources for completing advance directives, including links to each State's advance directive forms.

Driving Safety

Recommending that a patient limit driving—or that a patient give up his or her driver's license—is one of the most difficult topics a doctor has to address. Because driving is associated with independence and identity, making the decision not to drive is very hard.

For more information on safe driving, contact

AAA Foundation for Traffic Safety
607 14th Street, NW, Suite 201
Washington, DC 20005
1-202-638-5944
www.seniordrivers.org

AARP
601 E Street, NW Washington, DC 20049
1-888-227-7669 (toll-free)
www.aarp.org/families/driver_safety
The AARP Driver Safety Program offers classes to help motorists over the age of 50 improve their driving skills.

American Association of Motor Vehicle Administrators
4301 Wilson Boulevard, Suite 400
Arlington, VA 22203
1-703-522-4200
www.granddriver.info

The American Association of Motor Vehicle Administrators sponsors a program designed to educate aging drivers and their caregivers.

American Medical Association (AMA)
5515 North State Street
Chicago, IL 60654
1-800-621-8335 (toll-free)
www.ama-assn.org/ama/pub/category/10791.html

The AMA offers guidance for physicians to address problems about driving and older adults. For details, download the *Physician's Guide to Assessing and Counseling Older Drivers* from the website.

As with other difficult subjects, try to frame it as a common concern of older patients. Mention, for instance, that aging can lead to slowed reaction times and impaired vision. In addition, it may be harder to move the head to look back, quickly turn the steering wheel, or safely hit the brakes. Ask the patient about any car accidents. When necessary, warn patients about medications that may make them sleepy or impair judgment. Also, a device such as an automatic defibrillator or pacemaker might cause irregular heartbeats or dizziness that can make driving dangerous. You might ask if she or he has thought about alternative transportation methods if driving is no longer an option.

Elder Abuse and Neglect

Be alert to the signs and symptoms of elder abuse. If you notice that a patient delays seeking treatment or offers improbable explanations for injuries, for example, you may want to bring up your concerns. The laws in most States require helping professionals, such as doctors and nurses, to report suspected abuse or neglect.

For more information on elder abuse, contact

National Center on Elder Abuse
Center for Community Research and Services University of Delaware
297 Graham Hall
Newark, DE 19716
1-302-831-3525
www.ncea.aoa.gov
This consortium of organizations provides information about and conducts research on elder abuse.

Older people caught in an abusive situation are not likely to say what is happening to them for fear of reprisal or because of diminished cognitive abilities. If you suspect abuse, ask about it in a constructive, compassionate tone. If the patient lives with a family caregiver, you might start by saying that caregiver responsibilities can cause a lot of stress. Stress sometimes may cause caregivers to lose their temper. You can assist by recommending a support group or alternative arrangements (such as respite care). Give the patient opportunities to bring up this concern, but if necessary, raise the issue yourself.

End-of-Life Care

Most older people have thought about the prospect of their own death and are willing to discuss their wishes regarding end-of-life care. You can help ease some of the discomfort simply by being willing to talk about dying and by being open to discussions about these important issues and concerns. It may be helpful to do this early in your relationship with the patient when discussing medical and family history. Stay alert to cues that the patient may want to talk about this subject again. Encourage the patient to discuss end- of-life decisions early with family members and to consider a living will.

For more information on end-of-life care, contact

Education in Palliative and End-of-life Care (EPEC)
Northwestern University, Feinberg School of Medicine

750 North Lake Shore Drive, Suite 601
Chicago, IL 60611
1-312-503-3087
www.epec.net
EPEC provides physicians the basic knowledge and skills needed to care for dying patients.

National Hospice and Palliative Care Organization
1731 King Street, Suite 100
Alexandria, VA 22314
1-800-658-8898 (toll-free)
1-877-658-8896 (toll-free, multilingual helpline)
www.nhpco.org
NHPCO links to care organizations and the consumer website, www.caringinfo.org.

Of course, it is not always easy to determine who is close to death; even experienced clinicians find that prognostication can be difficult. Even if you have already talked with your patient about end-of-life concerns, it still can be hard to know the right time to re-introduce this issue. Some clinicians find it helpful to ask themselves, *"Would I be surprised if Mr. Flowers were to die this year?"* If the answer is "no," then it makes sense to start working with the patient and family to address end-of-life concerns, pain and symptom management, home health, and hospice care. You can offer to help patients review their advance directives. Include these updates in your medical records to ensure that patients receive the care they want.

Financial Barriers

Rising health care costs make it difficult for some people to follow treatment regimens. Your patients may be too embarrassed to mention their financial concerns. Studies have shown that many clinicians also are reluctant to bring up costs. If possible, designate an administrative staff person with a good bedside manner to discuss money and payment questions. This person can also talk with your patient about changes in Medicare and the Part D prescription drug coverage plans.

For more information on financial assistance, contact

Medicare Rights Center
520 Eighth Avenue, North Wing, 3rd Floor
New York, NY 10018
1-212-869-3850
1224 M Street, NW, Suite 100
Washington, DC 20005
1-202-637-0961
Main number: 1-800-333-4114 (toll-free)
www.medicarerights.org
The toll-free consumer hotline provides free counseling services about Medicare, including the prescription drug benefit.

National Council on Aging
www.benefitscheckup.org
The Council's online resource offers a searchable list of programs that can help with health care costs.

Partnership for Prescription Assistance
1-888-477-2669 (toll-free)
www.pparx.org
Many pharmaceutical companies offer reduced medication fees for patients who meet income requirements and other criteria. The website has a directory of prescription drug patient assistance programs.

The resources in this section may help when you talk with your patients about their financial concerns. In addition, your State Health Insurance Assistance Program (SHIP) may be helpful.

Long-Term Care

Long-term care includes informal caregiving, assisted living, home health services, adult day care, nursing homes, and community-based programs.

Early in your relationship with an older patient, you can begin to talk about the possibility that he or she may eventually require long-term care of some kind. By raising this topic, you are helping your patient think about what he or she might need in the future and how to plan for those needs. For instance, you might talk about what sort of assistance you think your patient will need, how soon in the future he or she will need the extra help, and where he or she might get this assistance.

For more information on long-term care, contact

> **Nursing Home Compare**
> www.medicare.gov/nhcompare/home.asp
> Medicare provides an online resource with detailed information about the past performance of every Medicare- and Medicaid-certified nursing home in the country.
>
> **Eldercare Locator**
> 1-800-677-1116 (toll-free)
> www.eldercare.gov
> The Eldercare Locator offers referrals to and information on services for seniors.

Mental Health

Despite many public campaigns to educate people about mental health and illness, there is still a stigma attached to mental health problems. Some older adults may find mental health issues difficult to discuss.

Such conversations, however, can be lifesavers. Primary care doctors have a key opportunity to recognize when a patient is depressed and/or suicidal. In fact, 70 percent of older patients who commit suicide have seen a primary care physician within the previous month. This makes it especially important for you to be alert to the signs and symptoms of depression.

As with other subjects, try a general approach to bringing up mental health concerns. For example, *"A lot of us develop sleep problems as we get older, but this can be a sign of depression, which sometimes we can treat."* Because older adults may have atypical symptoms, it is important to listen closely to what your patient has to say about trouble sleeping, lack of energy, and general aches and pains. It is easy to dismiss these as "just aging" and leave depression undiagnosed and therefore untreated.

For more information on mental health, contact

American Association for Geriatric Psychiatry
7910 Woodmont Avenue, Suite 1050
Bethesda, MD 20814-3004
1-301-654-7850
www.aagponline.org
The Association promotes the mental health and well-being of older people and works to improve the care of those with late-life mental disorders.

National Institute of Mental Health (NIMH)
6001 Executive Boulevard, Room 8184, MSC 9663
Bethesda, MD 20892-9663
1-866-615-6464 (toll-free)
1-866-415-8051 (TTY/toll-free)
www.nimh.nih.gov
NIMH, part of the National Institutes of Health, funds and conducts mental health research and distributes information to health professionals and the public.

Sexuality

An understanding, accepting attitude can help promote a more comfortable discussion of sexuality. Try to be sensitive to verbal and other cues. Don't assume that an older patient is no longer sexually active, does not care about sex, or necessarily is heterosexual. In fact, research has found that a majority of older Americans are sexually active and view intimacy as an important part of life. Depending on indications earlier in the interview, you may decide to approach the subject directly (for example, *"Are you satisfied with your sex life?"*) or more obliquely with allusions to changes that sometimes occur in marriage. If appropriate, follow up on patient cues. You might note that patients sometimes have concerns about their sex life and then wait for a response. It is also effective to share anonymous anecdotes about a person in a similar situation or to raise the issue in the context of physical findings (for example, *"Some people taking this medication have trouble . . .*

Have you experienced anything like that?"). Don't forget to talk with your patient about the importance of safe sex. For example, *"It's been a while since your husband died. If you are considering dating again, would you like to talk about how to have safe sex?"* Any person, regardless of age, who is not in a long-term relationship with a faithful partner and has unprotected sex, is at risk of sexually transmitted disease.

For more information on sexuality, contact

>**Centers for Disease Control and Prevention**
>1600 Clifton Road
>Atlanta, GA 30333
>1-800-232-4636 (toll-free)
>www.cdc.gov/hiv/topics/over50

>**Mayo Foundation for Medical Education and Research**
>www.mayoclinic.com/health/sexual-health/HA00035
>This website has articles about sexual health and sexuality for adults age 50 and older.

>**Sexuality Information and Education Council of the United States**
>90 John Street, Suite 402
>New York, NY 10038
>1-212-819-9770 www.siecus.org

Spirituality

For some older people, spirituality takes on new meaning as they age or face serious illness. By asking patients about their religious and spiritual practices, you can learn something about their health care choices and preferences. How a patient views the afterlife can sometimes help in framing the conversation.

For example, some patients feel that their fate is in the hands of a higher power, and this may prevent them from making treatment decisions. For patients who report suffering and distress about illness or end-of-life, a referral to a hospital or nursing home chaplain may be helpful.

For more information on spirituality, contact

>**Association of Professional Chaplains**
>1701 East Woodfield Road, Suite 400
>Schaumburg, IL 60173
>1-847-240-1014
>www.professionalchaplains.org

The Association is an interfaith professional society providing education, research, and certification for its members and web links to many chaplaincy organizations.

>**George Washington University Institute for Spirituality and Health**
>2300 K Street, NW, Suite 313
>Washington, DC 20037-1898
>1-202-994-6220
>www.gwish.org

The Institute recognizes spiritual dimensions of health. Its work focuses on bringing increased attention to the spiritual needs of patients, families, and health care professionals.

Clinicians have found that very direct and simple questions are the best way to broach this subject. You might start, for instance, by asking, *"What has helped you to deal with challenges in the past?"*

Substance Abuse

Alcohol and drug abuse are major public health problems, even for older adults. Sometimes people can become dependent on alcohol or other drugs as they confront the challenges of aging, even if they did not have a problem when younger. Because baby boomers have a higher rate of lifetime substance abuse than did their parents, the number of people in this age group needing treatment is likely to grow.

For more information on substance abuse, contact

>**National Clearinghouse for Alcohol and Drug Information (NCADI)**

P.O. Box 2345
Rockville, MD 20847-2345
1-800-729-6686 (toll-free)
www.health.org

NCADI, funded by the Substance Abuse and Mental Health Services Administration, is a one-stop resource for information on substance abuse prevention and addiction treatment.

One approach you might try is to mention that some medical conditions can become more complicated as a result of alcohol and other drug use. Another point to make is that alcohol and other drugs can increase the side effects of medication, or even reduce the medicine's effectiveness. From this starting point, you may find it easier to talk about alcohol or other drug use.

Urinary Incontinence

About 17 percent of men and 38 percent of women age 60 and older suffer from urinary incontinence. Several factors can contribute to incontinence.

For more information on urinary incontinence, contact

American Urological Association Foundation
1000 Corporate Boulevard
Linthicum, MD 21090
1-800-828-7866 (toll-free)
www.urologyhealth.org

The Foundation provides information on the prevention, detection, management, and cure of urologic diseases.

National Institute of Diabetes and Digestive and Kidney Diseases (NIDDK)
3 Information Way
Bethesda, MD 20892-3580
1-800-891-5390 (toll-free)
1-866-569-1162 (TTY/toll-free)
www.kidney.niddk.nih.gov

NIDDK, part of the National Institutes of Health, distributes publications on urinary incontinence and provides links to resources and support groups.

The Simon Foundation for Continence
P.O. Box 815
Wilmette, IL 60091
1-800-237-4666 (toll-free)
www.simonfoundation.org

The Foundation provides information about cure, treatment, and management techniques for incontinence.

Childbirth, infection, certain medications, and some illnesses are examples. Incontinence may go untreated because patients are embarrassed to mention it. Be sure to ask specifically about the problem. Try the "some people" approach: *"When some people cough or sneeze, they leak urine. Have you had this problem?"* You may want to explain that incontinence can often be significantly improved through bladder training; medication and surgery can also be effective treatments for certain types of incontinence.

In Summary

- Introduce sensitive topics with the "common concern" approach: *"As we age, many of us have more trouble with . . ."* or *"Some people taking this medication have trouble with . . ."*
- Keep educational materials available and visible to encourage discussion.
- Raise topics such as safe driving, long-term care, advance care directives, and end-of-life care early, before they become urgent matters.

SUPPORTING PATIENTS WITH CHRONIC CONDITIONS

Case managers can play an important role in educating patients and families and can connect them with appropriate community resources and services.

> **"Let's discuss living with . . ."**
>
> Four years ago, Mrs. Smoley suffered a stroke. Although she takes her pills just like the doctor ordered, she has not been able to quit smoking. Now she has emphysema and may soon need oxygen. Dr. Nguyen thinks she should participate in a disease management program at a local hospital that will give her the information she needs to manage on her own. "It could help you prevent the problems you've had with shortness of breath," the doctor explains. "And you might learn some tips about how to manage your day so that you have some more energy." She offers to help Mrs. Smoley schedule her first appointment.

Approximately 80 percent of older adults have at least one chronic health condition, and 50 percent have at least two chronic conditions. For many older people, coping with multiple chronic conditions is a real challenge. Learning to manage a variety of treatments while maintaining quality of life can be problematic. People with chronic conditions may have different needs, but they also share common challenges with other older adults, such as paying for care or navigating the complexities of the health care system.

Try to start by appreciating that people living with chronic disease are often living with loss—the loss of physical function, independence, or general well-being. Empathize with patients who feel angry, sad, lost, or bewildered. Ask, *"Is it hard for you to live with these problems?"* From there you can refer patients to community resources that may meet their needs or, when available, recommend a disease management program or case managers in the community.

Educating the Patient

Most older patients want to understand their medical conditions and are interested in learning how to manage them. Likewise, family members and other caregivers want this information. Physicians typically underestimate how much patients want to know and overestimate how long they spend giving information to patients. Devoting more attention to educating patients may seem like a luxury, but in the long run it can improve patients' adherence to treatment, increase patients' well-being, and save you time.

The following tips can help you inform patients and their caregivers about medical conditions and their treatment.

- Doctors' advice generally receives greatest credence, so the doctor should introduce treatment plans. Other medical team members have an important role, including building on the original instructions.
- Let your patient know you welcome questions. Indicate whom on your staff he or she can call to have questions answered later.
- Remember that some patients won't ask questions even if they want more information. Be aware of this tendency and think about making information available even if it is not requested.
- Provide information through more than one channel. In addition to talking to the patient, you can use fact sheets, drawings, models, videotapes, or audiotapes. In many cases, referrals to websites and support groups can be helpful.
- Encourage the patient or caregiver to take notes. It's helpful to offer a pad and pencil. Active involvement in recording information may promote your patient's retention and adherence.
- Repeat key points about the health problem and treatment at every office visit.
- Check that the patient and his or her caregivers understand what you say. One good approach is to ask that they repeat the main message in their own words.
- Provide encouragement. Call attention to strengths and ideas for improvement. Remember to provide continued reinforcement for new treatment or lifestyle changes.

Explaining Diagnoses

Clear explanations of diagnoses are critical. Uncertainty about a health problem can be upsetting. When patients do not understand their medical conditions, they tend not to follow the treatment plans.

In explaining diagnoses, it is helpful to begin by finding out what the patient believes is wrong, what the patient thinks will happen, and how much more he or she wants to know. Based on the patient's responses, you can correct any misconceptions and provide appropriate types of information.

Discussing Treatment

Some older patients may refuse treatment because they do not understand what it involves or how it will improve their health. In some cases, they may be frightened about side effects or have misinformation from friends and relatives with similar health problems. They may also be concerned about the cost of the treatment.

Treatment can involve lifestyle changes (such as diet and exercise) as well as medication. Make sure you develop and communicate treatment plans with the patient's input and consent. Tell the patient what to expect from the treatment, including recommended lifestyle change, what degree of improvement is realistic, and when he or she may start to feel better.

Keep medication plans as simple and straightforward as possible. For example, minimize the number of doses per day. Tailor the plan to the patient's situation and lifestyle, and try to reduce disruption to the patient's routine. Indicate the purpose of each medication. Make it clear which medications must be taken and on what schedule. It is helpful to say which drugs the patient should take only when having particular symptoms.

After proposing a treatment plan, check with the patient about its feasibility and acceptability. Work through what the patient feels may be obstacles to maintaining the plan. Try to resolve any misunderstandings. For example, make it clear that a referral to another doctor does not mean you are abandoning the patient. Provide oral and written instructions. Do not assume that all of your patients are able to read. Make sure the print is large enough for the patient to read.

Encourage your patient and his or her caregivers to take an active role in discovering how to manage chronic problems. Think in terms of joint problem solving or collaborative care. Such an approach can increase the patient's satisfaction while decreasing demands on your time.

In Summary

- The physician should provide key information and advice for greatest impact; other team members can build on that.
- To explain diagnoses, start by asking the patient what he or she understands and how much more he or she wants to know.

- After proposing a treatment plan, check with the patient on feasibility and acceptability; confirm that the patient understands the plan.
- Encourage the patient and caregivers to take an active role in managing a chronic problem.

BREAKING BAD NEWS

Delivering bad news is never easy, but tested strategies can ease the process.

> **"I wish I had better news."**
>
> Since Dr. Callas got Mrs. Larson's test results, he had been thinking about how to tell her she has Parkinson's disease. Because he didn't want to feel pressured for time, Dr. Callas made sure Mrs. Larson had today's last appointment. He knew she'd have a lot of questions. Knowing that Mrs. Larson suspected something was seriously wrong, Dr. Callas decided the best approach was to be gentle, but direct. He reviewed her chart for details, took a deep breath, and opened the exam room door . . .

Knowing how to communicate bad news can help you to make the process more bearable for patients. The Education in Palliative and End-of-Life Care Project (EPEC), www.epec.net, offers a module, "Communicating Bad News," that provides a practical approach. It indicates that breaking bad news in a compassionate yet direct way can help physicians and patients. And, although some of the advice may seem obvious, it may also be the sort of thing that is easily overlooked.

The first step is to prepare yourself. Before meeting with the patient, think about what you want to say and make sure that you have all of the information you need. Be sure there is enough time, rather than trying to schedule it between other appointments. If possible, ask your staff to hold calls and pages until the appointment is over.

You may feel more comfortable by first finding out what the patient knows about his or her condition. You might ask questions such as, *"Have you been worried about your illness or symptoms?"*

Next, you might spend a few moments finding out how much the patient really wants to know. Depending on their cultural background, personal history, or medical status, people may have different expectations and preferences for what they should be told. You might ask the patient if he or she wants to hear the prognosis, for example, or would prefer not to know.

If a patient's family has reservations about having the patient know the prognosis, you might ask them about their concerns. Legally, of course, you are obligated to tell the patient; however, you may negotiate some elements with the family. If you cannot resolve it, an ethics consultation may be helpful.

When you are ready to share the bad news, try to be as straightforward as possible, without speaking in a monotone or delivering a monologue. Be positive, but avoid the natural temptation to minimize the seriousness of the diagnosis. Communications experts suggest that you not start by saying, *"I'm sorry..."* Instead, try saying, *"I feel bad to have to tell you..."* After you have explained the bad news, you can express genuine sadness while reassuring the patient that you and others will be there to help.

Of course, people will respond differently to bad news; shock, anger, sorrow, despair, denial, blame, disbelief, and guilt all are common reactions. In some cases, people may simply have to leave the office. Try to give the patient and family time—and privacy—to react.

A good way to end this visit is to establish a plan for next steps. This may include gathering more information, ordering more tests, or preparing advance directives. Reassure the patient and family that you are not going to abandon them, regardless of referrals to other health care providers. Let them know how they can reach you—and be sure to respond when they call.

In follow-up appointments or conversations, give the patient an opportunity to talk again about the situation. Ask if he or she has more questions or needs help talking with family members or others about the diagnosis. Assess the patient's level of emotional distress and consider a referral to a mental health provider.

THE LANGUAGE OF BAD NEWS: PHRASES THAT HELP

These phrases can help you to be straightforward, yet compassionate:

Delivering Bad News

- "I'm afraid the news is not good. The biopsy showed you have colon cancer."

- "Unfortunately, there is no question about the results. You have emphysema."
- "The report is back, and it's not as we had hoped. It confirms that you have the early stages of Parkinson's disease."

Responding to Patient Reactions

- "I imagine this is difficult news."
- "Does this news frighten you?"
- "I wish the news were different."
- "Is there anyone you'd like me to call?"
- "I'll try to help you."
- "I'll help you tell your children."

Dealing with Prognosis

- "What are you expecting to happen?"
- "What would you like to have happen?"
- "How specific would you like me to be?"
- "What are your fears about what might happen?"

Adapted from: Emanuel LL, von Gunten CF, Ferris FF, and Hauser JM, eds. "Module 2: Communicating Bad News," The Education in Palliative and End-of-Life Care (EPEC) Curriculum: © The EPEC Project, 1999, 2003.

REFERRING PATIENTS TO CLINICAL TRIALS

Carefully conducted clinical trials are the primary way researchers find out if a promising treatment is safe and effective. Patients who participate in clinical research can gain access to new treatments before they are widely available and help others by contributing to medical research findings. Clinicians have an important role in continuing to care for patients who participate in clinical trials. Most trials offer short-term treatments related to a specific illness or condition. They do not provide extended or complete primary health care. You will continue your involvement in the patient's care but may need to communicate at times with your patient's clinical research team.

By working with the research team, you can ensure that other medications or treatment needed by your patient will not conflict with the protocol. For information about federally and privately supported clinical research, visit: www.clinicaltrials.gov

In Summary

- Prepare yourself for delivering bad news—allow enough time, and have calls held.
- Find out how much the patient understands and how much he or she wants to know about the prognosis.
- Be straightforward and compassionate.
- Give the patient time to react.
- Establish a plan for next steps; let the patient and family know you are not going to abandon them.
- Give the patient an opportunity to continue the conversation in follow-up appointments or calls.

WORKING WITH DIVERSE OLDER PATIENTS

Appreciating the richness of cultural and ethnic backgrounds among older patients and providing interpretation for those with limited English can help to promote good health care.

> **"Cultural differences, not divides."**
>
> Azeeza Houssani had been Dr. Smith's patient for several years. She had always carefully followed his instructions. So, Dr. Smith was surprised when Mrs. Houssani was not willing to take her morning medication with food, as directed. He reminded her that these drugs were very hard on the stomach and could cause her pain if taken without food. But Mrs. Houssani just shook her head. Rather than getting frustrated, Dr. Smith gently pursued her reasons.

> Mrs. Houssani explained that it was Ramadan and she could not eat or drink from sunrise to sunset. Dr. Smith thought a bit and suggested that she find out if it's okay to take medicine with food during Ramadan—there might be an exception for people in her situation who need to take medicine.

Understanding how different cultures view health care helps you to tailor questions and treatment plans to the patient's needs. Although you cannot become an expert in the norms and traditions of every culture, being sensitive to general differences can strengthen your relationship with your patients.

Each culture has its own rules about body language and interpretations of hand gestures. Some cultures point with the entire hand, because pointing with a finger is extremely rude behavior. For some cultures, direct eye contact is considered disrespectful. Until you are sure about a patient's background, you might opt for a conservative approach. And, if you aren't certain about a patient's preferences, ask.

The use of alternative medicines, herbal treatments, and folk remedies is common in many cultures. Be sure to ask your patient if he or she takes vitamins, herbal treatments, dietary supplements, or other alternative or complementary medicines. Also, in order to help build a trusting relationship, be respectful of native healers on whom your patient may also rely.

Older immigrants or non-native English speakers may need a medical interpreter. Almost 18 percent of the U.S. population speaks a language other than English at home, according to the Census Bureau. Among older people, 2.3 million report not speaking English or not speaking it very well. Federal policies require clinicians and health care providers who receive Federal funds, such as Medicare payments, to make interpretive services available to people with limited English.

Many clinicians rely on patients' family members or on the ad hoc services of bilingual staff members, but experts strongly discourage this practice and recommend the use of trained medical interpreters. Family members or office staff may be unable to interpret medical terminology, may inadvertently misinterpret information, or may find it difficult to relay bad news. Although a patient may choose to have a family member translate, the patient should be offered access to a professional interpreter.

For more information on working with patients with diverse cultural backgrounds, contact

Management Sciences for Health
784 Memorial Drive
Cambridge, MA 02139-4613
1-617-250-9500
http://erc.msh.org

This organization publishes *The Provider's Guide to Quality & Culture*. The *Guide* offers materials for health care providers who work with diverse populations, including information about common beliefs and practices.

National Institute on Aging (NIA) Information Center
P.O. Box 8057
Gaithersburg, MD 20898-8057
1-800-222-2225 (toll-free)
www.nia.nih.gov/espanol
www.nia.nih.gov/health

The NIA Spanish-language website provides accurate, up-to-date information in Spanish on a variety of health issues of interest to seniors. The website offers free publications and links to other health-related Spanish-language resources.

National Institutes of Health (NIH)
www.salud.nih.gov

The NIH has a wealth of patient education materials—a wide variety of which are available in Spanish. Visit the website for a complete list of Spanish-language resources.

National Library of Medicine MedlinePlus
www.medlineplus.gov/spanish

Office of Minority Health
P.O. Box 37337
Washington, DC 20013-7337

1-800-444-6472 (toll-free)
http://minorityhealth.hhs.gov

This Federal agency works to develop health policies and programs that help to eliminate racial and ethnic disparities in health.

When working with non-native English-speaking patients, be sure to ask which language they prefer to speak and whether or not they read and write English (and, if not, which language they do read). Whenever possible, offer patients appropriate translations of written material or refer them to bilingual resources. If translations are not available, ask the medical interpreter to translate medical documents.

FINDING A MEDICAL INTERPRETER

A number of States have associations and foundations that can help with locating, and in some cases provide funding for, medical interpreters. Some State Medicaid offices offer reimbursement for medical interpretation services. A web search can locate State organizations and local services. Or you can contact:

National Council on Interpreting in Health Care
5505 Connecticut Avenue, NW, #119
Washington, DC 20015-2601
1-202-596-2436
www.ncihc.org

In Summary

- Keep in mind that cultural differences have an impact on how patients view doctors and medicine.
- Ask about patients' use of alternative and complementary medicines.
- Use a professional medical interpreter rather than family members or untrained staff.
- Provide written materials in the patient's primary language.

INCLUDING FAMILIES AND CAREGIVERS

By communicating effectively with all the individuals involved in your patient's care, you can help him or her while also making efficient use of time and resources.

> **"What would you like your family to know?"**
>
> Dr. Hwang noticed that Mrs. Patrick wasn't getting her medication dosage quite right. Mrs. Patrick admitted that sometimes she does not remember everything prescribed for her to do. Dr. Hwang wondered if Mrs. Patrick should bring her daughter to her next appointment. Mrs. Patrick agreed, but at the following doctor visit she still came alone. Dr. Hwang was puzzled. When he asked her about it, Mrs. Patrick said that she was concerned her daughter wouldn't let her speak for herself and that she has some personal issues she'd like to discuss with him that she doesn't want her daughter to know about. Dr. Hwang assured her that he would keep her involved in the conversation about her health and that they could have some private time to discuss any personal matters. Next time, Mrs. Patrick brought her daughter to the visit.

Family and informal caregivers play an important role in the lives of their loved ones. They also play an increasingly important role in how the health care system functions.

Informal caregivers may be important "informants." They can also help to reinforce the importance of information you give or the treatment you prescribe.

To protect and honor patient privacy, be sure to check with the patient on how he or she sees the companion's role. In many cases, the caregiver or companion can be a facilitator, helping the patient express concerns and reinforcing what you say. But it is best not to assume that a companion should be included in the medical encounter. First, check with the patient. Conducting the physical exam alone protects the patient's privacy and allows you to raise sensitive issues. For instance, the best time to conduct a "mini-mental" test is during a private exam, so that a family member cannot answer questions or cover for the patient's cognitive lapses.

When a companion is present, be aware of communication issues that arise in three-party interactions. Whenever possible, try to sit so that you form a triangle and can address both the patient and companion face-to-face. Be careful not to direct your remarks to the companion. By not falling into this trap, you can prevent the encounter from feeling like a "two against one" match.

For more information on working with families and caregivers, contact

Administration on Aging (AoA)
Washington, DC 20201
1-202-619-0724
www.aoa.gov
AoA provides funds and community-based services for programs that serve older adults.

Eldercare Locator
1-800-677-1116 (toll-free)
www.eldercare.gov

The Eldercare Locator offers referrals to information on services for seniors.

Family Caregiver Alliance
180 Montgomery Street, Suite 900
San Francisco, CA 94104
1-800-445-8106 (toll-free)
www.caregiver.org
The Alliance offers programs to provide information to and support for caregivers.

National Alliance for Caregiving
4720 Montgomery Lane, 2nd Floor
Bethesda, MD 20814
www.caregiving.org
The National Alliance offers support and resources for the public and professionals.

National Family Caregivers Association
10400 Connecticut Avenue, Suite 500
Kensington, MD 20895-3944
1-800-896-3650 (toll-free)
www.nfcacares.org

This Association supports family caregivers and offers education, information, and referrals.

Families may want to make decisions for a loved one. Adult children especially may want to step in for a parent who has cognitive impairments. If a family member has been named the health care agent or proxy, under some circumstances, he or she has the legal authority to make care decisions. However, without this authority, the patient is responsible for making his or her own choices. Try to set clear boundaries with family members, and encourage others to respect them.

Family caregivers face many emotional, financial, and physical challenges. They often provide help with household chores, transportation, and personal care. More than one-third also give medications, injections, and medical treatments to the person for whom they care. It makes sense to view informal caregivers as "hidden patients" and be alert for signs of illness and stress. Caregivers may find it hard to make time for themselves. Encourage them to seek respite care so that they can recharge and take a break from the loved one. And remember, your encouragement and praise can help to sustain a caregiver.

In Summary

- Check with the patient on how he or she would like any family members or companions to participate in the medical encounter.
- Address the patient—try to avoid talking only to the family member or companion.
- Make it clear that the patient should make his or her own decisions unless legal authority to do so has been granted to someone else.
- Be alert to family caregivers' own health needs, including signs of stress.

Talking With Patients About Cognitive Problems

Communicating with a confused patient holds special challenges. Specific techniques can help health care providers to talk with patients and caregivers about a diagnosis.

> **"You mentioned having trouble with your memory."**
>
> Jonathan Jones had always been a meticulously organized man. His bills were paid on time; his car gas tank was always at least half full. He could be counted on to arrive slightly early for every appointment. Dr. Ross knew all this because he'd been taking care of the Jones family for nearly 30 years. So when Mr. Jones missed two appointments in a row, Dr. Ross knew something was not right and called him at home. The phone rang for quite a while before Mr. Jones answered, "Yes? Hello, Dr. Ross. Why are you calling? I don't have an appointment scheduled with you." The conversation added to Dr. Ross's concerns. The doctor made a note on the chart—it was time to broach the subject of memory loss with Mr. Jones. After so many years, this was going to be a hard discussion.

Cognitive Impairment

Aging itself can cause deficits in cognition that vary from person to person. While some older people show little or no decrease in cognitive function, others may be very worried about their memory and may fear dementing disorders such as Alzheimer's disease (AD). But, not all cognitive problems are caused by AD. Various illnesses, both physical and mental, can cause temporary, reversible cognitive impairment. Certain drug combinations can also cause a problem.

Identifying and working with older adults who have cognitive impairment are important for their safety and for the safety of others. Older patients with cognitive impairment can develop difficulties in remembering and correctly adhering to instructions about medications for their other health problems. In addition, activities such as cooking and driving can become dangerous.

Many patients with cognitive impairments experience behavioral changes. For instance, they may withdraw from or lose interest in activities, grow irritable or uncharacteristically angry when frustrated or tired, or become insensitive to other people's feelings. During more advanced stages of cognitive impairment, people may behave inappropriately—kicking, hitting, screaming, or cursing. Depending on the stage of the disease, you can suggest activities that your patient might still enjoy—for example, listening to music and perhaps dancing, playing games, gardening, or spending time with pets.

Some of your older patients may have a specific condition called mild cognitive impairment (MCI). People with MCI have ongoing memory problems but do not have other losses associated with AD such as confusion, attention problems, or difficulty with language. Some people's cognitive problems may not get worse for many years. Some people with MCI may convert to AD over time. Research is ongoing to determine better which people with MCI will develop AD.

The suggestions in this section of the booklet pertain specifically to effective communication with patients with cognitive impairments.

Diagnosis

Accurate diagnosis of AD or other cognitive problems can help your older patient and his or her family to plan for the future. Early diagnosis offers the best chance to treat the symptoms of the disease, when possible, and to discuss ways of positively coping with the condition, including discussing care options. A relatively early diagnosis allows patients to make financial plans, prepare advance directives, and express informed consent for research. Yet data suggest that only a small fraction of people with AD are ever diagnosed.

When patients are only mildly impaired, they can be adept at covering up what is happening to them. However, giving a few straightforward tests, using a medical history, and taking a family history from another family member can often tell you if there are persistent or worsening problems. It is best to conduct tests or interviews with the patient alone so that family members or companions cannot prompt the patient. Information can also be gleaned from the patient's behavior on arrival in your office or from telephone interactions with staff. Family members who may contact you in advance or following the visit are also a source of information, but keep in mind patient privacy concerns.

Although assessing an older person's cognitive function is important, formal testing of mental status tends to provoke anxiety. If you are concerned about a patient's cognition, it might be best to leave any formal testing of mental status until the latter part of the appointment—either between the history and the physical examination or after the examination—or to refer the patient to a neuropsychologist for more detailed assessment of cognition. If you administer a cognitive status test, try to present it in the context of concerns the patient has expressed. Providing support and encouragement during the testing can decrease stress.

There are limitations to any mental status test—for example, the test results can reflect level of education, or the results may appear normal early in the disease. The most commonly used screen is the Mini-Mental State Examination. This test can be used to screen patients for cognitive impairment and can be administered in the primary care setting in about 10 minutes. A positive finding suggests the need for referral to a neurologist or neuropsychologist for a more detailed diagnosis.

Cognitive impairment may reflect a variety of conditions, some reversible. In particular, it is important to review your patient's medications to check for anticholinergic or other potentially inappropriate medications. However, since patients or caregivers may assume that the cause is Alzheimer's disease, you may need to explain the need for a careful history, laboratory tests, and physical examination to search for other conditions or issues.

If your patient does have mild to moderate cognitive impairment, you might ask if there is someone who helps when he or she has trouble remembering. If your patient says yes, you could also ask if it would be a good idea for you to discuss the patient's treatment plans with the helper and keep his or her name in your notes for future reference. Make these arrangements early, and check that the patient has given you formal authorization to include the helper in the conversation about your patient's care.

For more information on Alzheimer's disease, contact

Alzheimer's Association
225 North Michigan Avenue, Floor 17
Chicago, IL 60601-7633
1-800-272-3900 (toll-free)
www.alz.org

This national voluntary health organization supports Alzheimer's disease research and care and offers information and support to patients and families. It has local chapters with community information including referrals, support groups, and safety services.

Alzheimer's Disease Education and Referral (ADEAR) Center
P.O. Box 8250
Silver Spring, MD 20907-8250
1-800-438-4380 (toll-free)
www.nia.nih.gov/alzheimers

A service of NIA, ADEAR provides information, publications, referrals, a health information database, and a clinical trials database for the public and for health care professionals.

For updated Alzheimer's disease diagnostic guidelines: www.nia.nih.gov/ alzheimers/resources/diagnosticguidelines.htm

Alzheimer's Foundation of America
322 8th Avenue, 7th Floor
New York, NY 10001
1-866-232-8484 (toll-free)
www.alzfdn.org

The Foundation brings together groups around the country, including assisted living organizations, community services agencies, State agencies, and others, to collaborate on education, resources, and program design and implementation for people with AD, their caregivers, and families.

Conveying Findings

Some patients may prefer a cautious, reserved explanation. You might consider saying something like, *"You have a memory disorder, and I believe it will get worse as time goes on. It's not your fault. It may not help for you to try harder. Now is probably a good time for you to start making financial and legal plans before your memory and thinking get worse."* Some patients may prefer more precise language and appreciate it when a doctor uses specific words like Alzheimer's disease. If possible, schedule additional time for the appointment so that you can listen and respond to the patient's or caregiver's concerns. Also, if possible, offer to have a follow-up appointment to further discuss what to expect from the diagnosis.

Regardless of how you present the diagnosis, providing written materials can make a big difference in helping your patient and his or her family know what to expect. The NIA's Alzheimer's Disease Education and Referral (ADEAR) Center has free publications you can include in a patient/caregiver information packet. You might want to refer your patient to a neurologist or neuropsychologist for testing. The Alzheimer's Association or other supportive organizations can provide assistance in planning, social services, and care.

COMMUNICATING WITH A CONFUSED PATIENT

- Try to address the patient directly, even if his or her cognitive capacity is diminished.
- Gain the person's attention. Sit in front of him or her and maintain eye contact.
- Speak distinctly and at a natural rate of speed. Resist the temptation to speak loudly.
- Help orient the patient. Explain (or re-explain) who you are and what you will be doing.
- If possible, meet in surroundings familiar to the patient. Consider having a family member or other familiar person present at first.
- Support and reassure the patient. Acknowledge when responses are correct.
- If the patient gropes for a word, gently provide assistance.
- Make it clear that the encounter is not a "test," but rather a search for information to help the patient.
- Use simple, direct wording. Present one question, instruction, or statement at a time.
- If the patient hears you but does not understand you, rephrase your statement.
- Although open-ended questions are advisable in most interview situations, patients with cognitive impairments often have difficulty coping with them. Consider using a yes-or-no or multiple-choice format.
- Remember that many older people have hearing or vision problems, which can add to their confusion.
- Consider having someone call the patient to follow up on instructions after outpatient visits.
- If the patient can read, provide written instructions and other background information about the problem and options for solutions.

Informing family members or others that the patient may have Alzheimer's disease or any cognitive impairment may be done in a family conference or group meeting, which should be arranged with the consent of the patient. In some situations, a series of short visits may be more suitable. You should make clear you will continue to be available for care, information, guidance, and support. If you are unable to provide all of these services, it would make a tremendous difference if you could refer the patient and family to a service organization.

Working with Family Caregivers

All family caregivers face challenges, but these challenges are compounded for people caring for patients with Alzheimer's disease and other dementias. The patient usually declines slowly, over the course of several years. This is an exhausting and disturbing experience for everyone. The following suggestions are especially useful for family caregivers in these situations:

- Persuade caregivers to get regular respite, especially when patients require constant attention. Ask if the caregiver, who is at considerable risk for stress-related disorders, is receiving adequate health care.
- Explain that much can be done to improve the patient's quality of life. Measures, such as modifications in daily routine and medications for anxiety, depression, or sleep, may help control symptoms.
- Let the caregivers know there is time to adapt. Decline is rarely rapid. Provide information about the consumer resources and support services available from groups.
- Help caregivers plan for the possibility that they eventually may need more help at home or may have to look into residential care.

In Summary

- Using a simple screen, such as the Mini-Mental State Examination, assess the patient's cognitive function when alone with him or her. Refer the patient to a specialist (e.g., neurologist or neuropsychologist) for diagnosis of cognitive impairment.
- Reassure the patient if there is no serious mental decline.

- Decide how to talk about serious cognitive problems, depending on how much the patient wants to know and can understand.
- Communicate with family members in a family conference, arranged with the patient's consent.
- Suggest activities that the patient and family might still enjoy.
- Be alert to caregivers' needs for information, resources, and respite.

KEEPING THE DOOR OPEN

> **"Effective Communication"**
>
> *Advising an older man about starting an exercise program . . . counseling a woman about the proper way to take her osteoporosis medication . . . discussing end-of-life care options with the family of a long-time older patient who is dying.* These are just some examples of the complex and sensitive issues facing clinicians who treat older people. Health care providers who communicate successfully with older patients may gain their trust and cooperation, enabling everyone to work as a team to handle physical and mental health problems that might arise. Effective communication techniques, like those discussed in this handbook, can save time, increase satisfaction for both patient and practitioner, and improve the provider's skill in managing the care of his or her patients.

Ongoing communication is key to working effectively with your older patient. If a patient does not follow recommendations or starts missing appointments, explore whether or not a difficulty in communication has developed. Paying attention to communication increases the odds of greater health for your patient and satisfaction for you both.

For resources on working with older patients, contact

National Institute on Aging (NIA)
Building 31, Room 5C27
31 Center Drive, MSC 2292
Bethesda, MD 20892
1-301-496-1752
www.nia.nih.gov

NIA funds research on the science of aging and provides information and materials for the public and for professionals. It is the primary Federal agency for Alzheimer's disease research and education.

For NIA publications:
National Institute on Aging Information Center
P.O. Box 8057
Gaithersburg, MD 20898-8097
1-800-222-2225 (toll-free)
1-800-222-4225 (TTY/toll-free)
www.nia.nih.gov/health

NIHSeniorHealth
www.nihseniorhealth.gov
This is a senior-friendly website from the National Institute on Aging and the National Library of Medicine that has health and wellness information for older adults. Special features make it simple to use. For example, you can click on a button to have the text read out loud or to make the type larger.

American Geriatrics Society (AGS)
40 Fulton Street, 18th Floor
New York, NY 10038
1-212-308-1414
www.americangeriatrics.org

AGS has programs in patient care, research, professional and public education, and public policy. The AGS website also offers many clinical resources, including:

- *Geriatrics At Your Fingertips*, a pocket-sized guide to caring for older patients
- *The Geriatric Review Syllabus*, featuring relevant online educational programs

American Medical Association (AMA)
515 North State Street
Chicago, IL 60654
1-800-621-8335 (toll-free)
www.ama-assn.org (search for "aging")

The AMA has several ongoing initiatives to address a variety of aging issues.

Gerontological Society of America (GSA)
1220 L Street, NW, Suite 901
Washington, DC 20005-4001
1-202-842-1275
www.geron.org

GSA is a non-profit, professional organization whose members include researchers, educators, practitioners, and policymakers.

PUBLICATIONS AT A GLANCE

The National Institute on Aging offers free publications you might use when talking with your older patients. You can order single or multiple copies from:

National Institute on Aging Information Center
P.O. Box 8057
Gaithersburg, MD 20898-9057
1-800-222-2225 (toll-free)
1-800-222-4225 (TTY/toll-free)
www.nia.nih.gov/health

NIA has free *AgePage* fact sheets on a variety of topics. Here is a selection of what's available. The asterisk (*) indicates those also available in Spanish.

Diseases/ Conditions	
	• *Arthritis Advice**
	• *Cancer Facts For People Over 50**
	• *Diabetes In Older People —A Disease You Can Manage**
	• *Hearing Loss**
	• *High Blood Pressure**
	• *Osteoporosis: The Bone Thief**
	• *Prostate Problems**
	• *Shingles**
	• *Stroke**

Safety	• Crime And Older People*
	• Falls And Fractures*
	• Medicines: Use Them Safely*
	• Older Drivers*
	• Online Health Information: Can You Trust It?
Wellness	• A Good Night's Sleep*
	• Aging And Your Eyes*
	• Concerned About Constipation?*
	• Dietary Supplements
	• Exercise and Physical Activity: Getting Fit for Life*
	• Flu Get the Shot*
	• Foot Care*
	• Healthy Eating After 50*
	• Hyperthermia: Too Hot for Your Health*
	• Hypothermia: A Cold Weather Hazard*
	• Shots for Safety*
	• Skin Care And Aging*
	• Smoking: It's Never Too Late To Stop*
	• Taking Care of Your Teeth and Mouth*
Other Subjects	• Alcohol Use In Older People*
	• Beware Of Health Scams*
	• Considering Surgery*
	• Depression*
	• Forgetfulness: Knowing When To Ask For Help*
	• Getting Your Affairs in Order
	• HIV, AIDS, and Older People*
	• Mourning the Death of a Spouse
	• Nursing Homes: Making The Right Choice*
	• Sexuality In Later Life*
	• Urinary Incontinence*
In-depth publications are also available. Examples are listed below.	
	• End of Life: Helping With Comfort and Care
	• Exercise and Physical Activity: Your Everyday Guide from the National Institute on Aging*
	• So Far way: Twenty Questions and Answers About Long-Distance Caregiving
	• Talking With Your Doctor: A Guide for Older People*
	• There's No Place Like Home—for Growing Old: Tips from the National Institute on Aging

NIA's ADEAR Center has a wide variety of free publications for people with cognitive problems, their families, and caregivers, such as *Understanding Alzheimer's Disease* and *Caring for a Person with Alzheimer's Disease*. To order, contact:

Alzheimer's Disease Education and Referral Center
P.O. Box 8250
Silver Spring, MD 20907-8250
1-800-438-4380 (toll-free)
www.nia.nih.gov/alzheimers

SERVICES AT A GLANCE

You want to help your patients get the services they need. But you may not be sure where to find the right resource. This is a starting place. We've identified some of the most common concerns and listed a few national resources that might be helpful.

What's the Problem?	What's a Solution?	Helpful Resources
Abuse/neglect	Mandatory reporting to adult protective services	**National Center on Elder Abuse** For your State Adult Protective Services: www.ncea.aoa.gov Call local police or 911, if serious situation
Caregiver assistance	Respite care	**National Respite Locator Service** www.respitelocator.org
Caregiving	Adult day care, nursing home care	**National Adult Day Services Association** 1-877-745-1440 (toll-free) www.nadsa.org **Nursing Home Compare service** www.medicare.gov/nhcompare/home.asp
Daily living assistance	Home health aide	**Eldercare Locator** 1-800-677-1116 (toll-free) www.eldercare.gov

What's the Problem?	What's a Solution?	Helpful Resources
Financial assistance	Case manager or supportive community programs	**National Council on Aging** To assess eligibility: www.benefitscheckup.org
Health information	Free fact sheets, booklets, and web resources	**National Institute on Aging Information Center** 1-800-222-2225 (toll-free) www.nia.nih.gov/health **NIH SeniorHealth** www.nihseniorhealth.gov **National Institutes of Health National Library of Medicine** www.medlineplus.gov
Household assistance	Homemaker assistant	**Eldercare Locator** 1-800-677-1116 (toll-free) www.eldercare.gov
Nutrition	Meals on Wheels or congregate meal sites	**Meals on Wheels Association of America** 1-703-548-5558 www.mowaa.org
Social support	Volunteer companions	**Eldercare Locator** 1-800-677-1116 (toll-free) www.eldercare.gov
Transportation	Medical transport benefits or other community programs	**National Association of Area Agencies on Aging** 1-202-872-0888 www.n4a.org **National Transit Hotline** 1-800-527-8279 (toll-free)
Utility costs	Utility subsidies	**National Energy Assistance Referral Project** 1-866-674-6327 (toll-free) http://liheap.ncat.org/profiles/energyhelp.htm

Chapter 2

TALKING WITH YOUR DOCTOR: A GUIDE FOR OLDER PEOPLE[*]

National Institute on Aging

OPENING THOUGHTS: WHY DOES IT MATTER?

How well you and your doctor talk to each other is one of the most important parts of getting good health care. But, talking to your doctor isn't always easy. It takes time and effort on your part as well as your doctor's.

In the past, the doctor typically took the lead and the patient followed. Today, a good patient- doctor relationship is more of a partnership. You and your doctor can work as a team, along with nurses, physician assistants, pharmacists, and other health care providers, to solve your medical problems and keep you healthy.

This means asking questions if the doctor's explanations or instructions are unclear, bringing up problems even if the doctor doesn't ask, and letting the doctor know if you have concerns about a particular treatment or change in your daily life. Taking an active role in your health care puts the responsibility for good communication on both you and your doctor.

---

[*] This is an edited, reformatted and augmented version of NIH Publication No. 05-3452, dated October 2005, reissued April 2010.

All of this is true at any age. But when you're older, it becomes even more important to talk often and comfortably with your doctor. That's partly because you may have more health conditions and treatments to discuss. It's also because your health has a big impact on other parts of your life, and that needs to be talked about too.

GETTING STARTED: CHOOSING A DOCTOR YOU CAN TALK TO

Finding a main doctor (often called your primary doctor or primary care doctor) that you feel comfortable talking to is the first step in good communication. It is also a way to ensure your good health. This doctor gets to know you and what your health is normally like. He or she can help you make medical decisions that suit your values and daily habits and can keep in touch with the other medical specialists and health care providers you may need.

If you don't have a primary doctor or are not at ease with the one you currently see, now may be the time to find a new doctor. Whether you just moved to a new city, changed insurance providers, or had a bad experience with your doctor or medical staff, it is worthwhile to spend time finding a doctor you can trust.

People sometimes hesitate to change doctors because they worry about hurting their doctor's feelings. But doctors understand that different people have different needs. They know it is important for everyone to have a doctor with whom they are comfortable.

Primary care doctors frequently are family practitioners, internists, or geriatricians. A geriatrician is a doctor who specializes in older people, but family practitioners and internists may also have a lot of experience with older patients.

The following suggestions can help you find a doctor who meets your needs:

Decide what you are looking for in a doctor — A good first step is to make a list of qualities that matter to you. Do you care if your doctor is a man or a woman? Is it important that your doctor has evening office hours, is associated with a specific hospital or medical center, or speaks your language? Do you prefer a doctor who has an individual practice or one who is part of a group so you can see one of your doctor's partners if your doctor is not available?

After you have made your list, go back over it and decide which qualities are most important and which are nice, but not essential.

Identify several possible doctors — Once you have a general sense of what you are looking for, ask friends and relatives, medical specialists, and other health professionals for the names of doctors with whom they have had good experiences. Rather than just getting a name, ask about the person's experiences. For example: say, *"What do you like about Dr. Smith?"* and *"Does this doctor take time to answer questions?"* A doctor whose name comes up often may be a strong possibility.

If you belong to a managed care plan—a health maintenance organization (HMO) or preferred provider organization (PPO)—you may be required to choose a doctor in the plan or else you may have to pay extra to see a doctor outside the network. Most managed care plans will provide information on their doctors' backgrounds and credentials. Some plans have websites with lists of participating doctors from which you can choose.

WHAT ARE HMOS AND PPOS?

Members of a health maintenance organization (HMO) pay a set monthly fee no matter how many (or few) times they see a doctor. Usually there are no deductibles or claims forms but you will have a co-payment for doctor visits and prescriptions. Each member chooses a primary care doctor from within the HMO network. The primary care doctor coordinates all care and, if necessary, refers members to specialists.

A preferred provider organization (PPO) is a network of doctors and other health care providers. The doctors in this network agree to provide medical services to PPO health plan members at discounted costs. Members can choose to see any doctor at any time. Choosing a non-PPO provider is called 'going out of network' and will cost more than seeing a member of the PPO network.

It may be helpful to develop a list of a few names you can choose from. As you find out more about the doctors on this list, you may rule out some of them. In some cases, a doctor may not be taking new patients and you may have to make another choice.

WHAT DOES "BOARD CERTIFIED" MEAN?

Doctors who are board certified have extra training after regular medical school. They also have passed an exam certifying their expertise in specialty areas. Examples of specialty areas are general internal medicine, family medicine, geriatrics, gynecology, and orthopedics. Board certification is one way to learn about a doctor's medical expertise; it doesn't tell you about the doctor's communication skills.

Consult reference sources — The *Directory of Physicians in the United States* and the *Official American Board of Medical Specialties Directory of Board Certified Medical Specialists* are available at many libraries. These books don't recommend individual doctors but they do provide a list of doctors you may want to consider. MedlinePlus, a website from the National Library of Medicine, has a comprehensive list of directories (www.nlm.nih.gov/medlineplus/ directories.html) which may also be helpful.

There are plenty of other Internet resources too—for example, you can find doctors through the American Medical Association's website at www.ama-assn.org (click on "Doctor Finder"). For a list of doctors who participate in Medicare, visit www.medicare.gov (click on "Search Tools" then "Find a Doctor"). WebMD also provides a list of doctors at www.webmd.com (click on "Doctors").

Don't forget to call your local or State medical society to check if complaints have been filed against any of the doctors you are considering.

Learn more about the doctors you are considering — Once you have narrowed your list to two or three doctors, call their offices. The office staff is a good source of information about the doctor's education and qualifications, office policies, and payment procedures. Pay attention to the office staff—you will have to deal with them often!

You may want to set up an appointment to meet and talk with a doctor you are considering. He or she is likely to charge you for such a visit. After the appointment, ask yourself whether this doctor is a person with whom you could work well. If you are not satisfied, schedule a visit with one of your other candidates.

When learning about a doctor, consider asking questions like:

- Do you have many older patients?
- How do you feel about involving my family in care decisions?
- Can I call or email you or your staff when I have questions? Do you charge for telephone or email time?
- What are your thoughts about complementary or alternative treatments?

When making a decision about which doctor to choose, you might want to ask yourself questions like:

- Did the doctor give me a chance to ask questions?
- Was the doctor really listening to me?
- Could I understand what the doctor was saying? Was I comfortable asking him or her to say it again?

Make a choice — Once you've chosen a doctor, make your first actual health care appointment. This visit may include a medical history and a physical exam. Be sure to bring your medical records, or have them sent from your former doctor. Bring a list of your current medicines or put the medicines in a bag and take them with you. If you haven't already met the doctor, ask for extra time during this visit to ask any questions you have about the doctor or the practice.

Summary: Choosing a Doctor You Can Talk To

- Decide what you are looking for in a doctor.
- Identify several possible doctors.
- Consult reference sources, including the Internet.
- Talk to office staff to learn more about the doctors you are considering.
- Make a choice.

Tips: What Do You Need to Know about a Doctor?

Basics

- Is the doctor taking new patients?
- Is the doctor covered by my insurance plan?
- Does the doctor accept Medicare?

Qualifications and Characteristics

- Is the doctor board certified? In what field?
- Is the age, sex, race, or religion of the doctor important?
- Will language be an obstacle to communication? Is there someone in the office who speaks my language?
- Do I prefer a group practice or an individual doctor?
- Does it matter which hospital the doctor admits patients to?

Logistics

- Is the location of the doctor's office important? How far am I willing to travel to see the doctor?
- Is there parking? What does it cost? Is the office on a bus or subway line?
- Does the building have an elevator? What about ramps for a wheelchair or walker?

Office Policies

- What days/hours does the doctor see patients?
- Are there times set aside for the doctor to take phone calls? Does the doctor accept emailed questions? Is there a charge for this service?
- Does the doctor ever make house calls?
- How far in advance do I have to make appointments?
- What's the process for urgent care? How do I reach the doctor in an emergency?
- Who takes care of patients after hours or when the doctor is away?

HOW SHOULD I PREPARE? GETTING READY FOR AN APPOINTMENT

A basic plan can help you make the most of your appointment whether you are starting with a new doctor or continuing with the doctor you've seen for years. The following tips will make it easier for you and your doctor to cover everything you need to talk about.

Make a list of your concerns and prioritize them —Make a list of what you want to discuss. For example, do you have a new symptom you want to ask the doctor about? Do you want to get a flu shot? Are you concerned about how a treatment is affecting your daily life? If you have more than a few items to discuss, put them in order and ask about the most important ones first. Don't put off the things that are really on your mind until the end of your appointment—bring them up right away!

Take information with you — Some doctors suggest you put all your prescription drugs, over-the-counter medicines, vitamins, and herbal remedies or supplements in a bag and bring them with you. Others recommend you bring a list of everything you take. You should also take your insurance cards, names, and phone numbers of other doctors you see, and your medical records if the doctor doesn't already have them.

Make sure you can see and hear as well as possible — Many older people use glasses or need aids for hearing. Remember to take your eyeglasses to the doctor's visit. If you have a hearing aid, make sure that it is working well and wear it. Let the doctor and staff know if you have a hard time seeing or hearing. For example, you may want to say: *"My hearing makes it hard to understand everything you're saying. It helps a lot when you speak slowly."*

Consider bringing a family member or friend —Sometimes it is helpful to bring a family member or close friend with you. Let your family member or friend know in advance what you want from your visit. Your companion can remind you what you planned to discuss with the doctor if you forget, she or he can take notes for you, and can help you remember what the doctor said.

Find an interpreter if you know you'll need one — If the doctor you selected or were referred to doesn't speak your language, consider bringing an interpreter with you. Sometimes community groups can help find an interpreter. Or you can call the doctor's office ahead of time to see if one can be provided for you. Sometimes doctors ask a staff member to help with interpretation. Even though some English-speaking doctors know basic medical terms in Spanish or other languages, you may feel more comfortable speaking in your own language, especially when it comes to sensitive subjects, such as sexuality or depression.

> ## RESOURCES IN SPANISH
>
> If you are looking for written information in Spanish there are an increasing number of resources that can help. For example, the National Institute on Aging (NIA) has translated many of its *AgePages* to Spanish. *AgePages* (called *Vivir Mejor la Tercera Edad* in Spanish) are short, easy-to-read fact sheets on a wide variety of health and aging topics. To get copies of these free publications you can call 1-800-222-2225; or order them online at www.nia.nih.gov/HealthInformation or www.nia.nih.gov/Espanol.

You can also ask a family member who speaks English to go with you. This person should be someone you trust with knowing your symptoms or condition. Finally, let the doctor, your interpreter, or the staff know if you do not understand your diagnosis or the instructions the doctor gives you. Don't let language barriers stop you from asking questions or voicing your concerns.

Plan to update the doctor — Let your doctor know what has happened in your life since your last visit. If you have been treated in the emergency room or by a specialist, tell the doctor right away. Mention any changes you have noticed in your appetite, weight, sleep, or energy level. Also tell the doctor about any recent changes in any medications you take or the effects they have had on you.

Summary: Getting Ready for an Appointment

- Be prepared: make a list of concerns.
- Take information with you.
- Make sure you can see and hear as well as possible.

FINDING AND USING AN INTERPRETER

- Look for an interpreter through community or neighborhood associations, the doctor's office staff, and your own network of friends and family.
- If possible, select someone with whom you will feel comfortable if they learn about your symptoms or condition. For example, you may not want to ask your children to interpret a conversation on sexuality.
- Consider telling your interpreter what you want to talk about with your doctor before the appointment.
- If your language is Spanish and your interpreter does not come from the same country or background as you, use universal Spanish terms to describe your symptoms.
- Make sure your interpreter understands your symptoms or condition before he or she conveys your message to the doctor. You don't want the doctor to prescribe the wrong medication!
- Don't be afraid to let your interpreter know if you did not understand something that was said, even if you need to ask that it be repeated several times.

- Consider bringing a family member or friend.
- Find an interpreter if you know you'll need one.
- Plan to update the doctor on what has happened since your last visit.

TIPS: GETTING STARTED WITH A NEW DOCTOR

Your first meeting is a good time to talk with the doctor and the office staff about some communication basics.

- **First name or last name** — When you see the doctor and office staff, introduce yourself and let them know by what name you like to be called. For example: *"Hello, my name is Mrs. Jones."* or *"Good morning, my name is Bob Smith. Please call me Bob."*
- **Ask how the office runs** — Learn what days are busiest and what times are best to call. Ask what to do if there is an emergency, or if you need a doctor when the office is closed.

- **Share your medical history** — Tell the doctor about your illnesses, operations, medical conditions, and other doctors you see. You may want to ask the doctor to send you a copy of the medical history form before your visit so you can fill it out at home where you have the time and information you need to complete it. If you have problems understanding how to fill out any of the forms, ask for help. Some community organizations provide this kind of help.
- **Share former doctors' names** — Give the new doctor all of your former doctors' names and addresses, especially if they are in a different city. This is to help your new doctor get copies of your medical records. Your doctor will ask you to sign a medical release form giving him or her permission to request your records.

WHAT CAN I SAY? GIVING INFORMATION

Talking about your health means sharing information about how you feel physically, emotionally, and mentally. Knowing how to describe your symptoms and bring up other concerns will help you become a partner in your health care.

Share any symptoms — A symptom is evidence of a disease or disorder in the body. Examples of symptoms include pain, fever, a lump or bump, unexplained weight loss or gain, or having a hard time sleeping.

Be clear and concise when describing your symptoms. Your description helps the doctor identify the problem. A physical exam and medical tests provide valuable information, but it is your symptoms that point the doctor in the right direction.

Questions to ask yourself about your symptoms:

- What exactly are my symptoms?
- Are the symptoms constant? If not, when do I experience them?
- Does anything I do make the symptoms better? Or worse?
- Do the symptoms affect my daily activities? Which ones? How?

Your doctor will ask when your symptoms started, what time of day they happen, how long they last (seconds? days?), how often they occur, if they seem to be getting worse or better, and if they keep you from going out or doing your usual activities.

Take the time to make some notes about your symptoms before you call or visit the doctor. Worrying about your symptoms is not a sign of weakness. Being honest about what you are experiencing doesn't mean that you are complaining. The doctor needs to know how you feel.

Give information about your medications — It is possible for medicines to interact causing unpleasant and sometimes dangerous side effects. Your doctor needs to know about ALL of the medicines you take, including over-the-counter (nonprescription) drugs and herbal remedies or supplements, so bring everything with you to your visit—don't forget about eye drops, vitamins, and laxatives. Tell the doctor how often you take each. Describe any drug allergies or reactions you have had. Say which medications work best for you. Be sure your doctor has the phone number of the pharmacy you use.

Tell the doctor about your habits — To provide the best care, your doctor must understand you as a person and know what your life is like. The doctor may ask about where you live, what you eat, how you sleep, what you do each day, what activities you enjoy, what your sex life is like, and if you smoke or drink. Be open and honest with your doctor. It will help him or her to understand your medical conditions fully and recommend the best treatment choices for you.

Voice other concerns — Your doctor may ask you how your life is going. This isn't being impolite or nosy. Information about what's happening in your life may be useful medically. Let the doctor know about any major changes or stresses in your life, such as a divorce or the death of a loved one. You don't have to go into detail; you may want to say something like: *"It might be helpful for you to know that my sister passed away since my last visit with you."* or *"I recently had to sell my home and move in with my daughter."*

Summary: Giving Information

- Share any symptoms.
- Give information about your medications.

- Tell the doctor about your habits.
- Voice other concerns.

> ## TIPS: MAKING GOOD USE OF YOUR TIME
>
> **Be honest** — It is tempting to say what you think the doctor wants to hear: for example, that you smoke less or eat a more balanced diet than you really do. While this is natural, it's not in your best interest. Your doctor can suggest the best treatment only if you say what is really going on. For instance, you might say: *"I have been trying to quit smoking, as you recommended, but I am not making much headway."*
>
> **Decide what questions are most important** — Pick three or four questions or concerns that you most want to talk about with the doctor. You can tell him or her what they are at the beginning of the appointment, and then discuss each in turn. If you have time, you can then go on to other questions.
>
> **Stick to the point** — Although your doctor might like to talk with you at length, each patient is given a limited amount of time. To make the best use of your time, stick to the point. For instance, give the doctor a brief description of the symptom, when it started, how often it happens, and if it is getting worse or better.
>
> **Share your point of view about the visit** — Tell the doctor if you feel rushed, worried, or uncomfortable. If necessary, you can offer to return for a second visit to discuss your concerns. Try to voice your feelings in a positive way. For example, you could say something like: *"I know you have many patients to see, but I'm really worried about this. I'd feel much better if we could talk about it a little more."*
>
> **Remember, the doctor may not be able to answer all your questions** — Even the best doctor may be unable to answer some questions. Most doctors will tell you when they don't have answers. They also may help you find the information you need or refer you to a specialist. If a doctor regularly brushes off your questions or symptoms as simply a part of aging, think about looking for another doctor.

WHAT CAN I ASK? GETTING INFORMATION

Asking questions is key to good communication with your doctor. If you don't ask questions, he or she may assume you already know the answer or that you don't want more information. Don't wait for the doctor to raise a specific question or subject because he or she may not know it's important to you. Be proactive. Ask questions when you don't know the meaning of a word (like aneurysm, hypertension, or infarct) or when instructions aren't clear (for example, does taking medicine with food mean before, during, or after a meal?).

Learn about medical tests — Sometimes doctors need to do blood tests, x rays, or other procedures to find out what is wrong or to learn more about your medical condition. Some tests, such as Pap smears, mammograms, glaucoma tests, and screenings for prostate and colorectal cancer, are done regularly to check for hidden medical problems.

Before having a medical test, ask your doctor to explain why it is important, what it will show, and what it will cost. Ask what kind of things you need to do to prepare for the test. For example, you may need to have an empty stomach, or you may have to provide a urine sample. Ask how you will be notified of the test results and how long they will take to come in.

Questions to ask about medical tests:

- Why is the test being done?
- What steps does the test involve? How should I get ready?
- Are there any dangers or side effects?
- How will I find out the results? How long will it take to get the results?
- What will we know after the test?

When the results are ready, make sure the doctor tells you what they are and explains what they mean. You may want to ask your doctor for a written copy of the test results. If the test is done by a specialist, ask to have the results sent to your primary doctor.

Discuss your diagnosis and what you can expect — A diagnosis identifies your disease or physical problem. The doctor makes a diagnosis based on the symptoms you are experiencing and the results of the physical exam, laboratory work, and other tests.

If you understand your medical condition, you can help make better decisions about treatment. If you know what to expect, it may be easier for you to deal with the condition.

Ask the doctor to tell you the name of the condition and why he or she thinks you have it. Ask how it may affect you and how long it might last. Some medical problems never go away completely. They can't be cured, but they can be treated or managed.

Questions to ask about your diagnosis:

- What may have caused this condition? Will it be permanent?
- How is this condition treated or managed? What will be the long-term effects on my life?
- How can I learn more about my condition?

Find out about your medications — Your doctor may prescribe a drug for your condition. Make sure you know the name of the drug and understand why it has been prescribed for you. Ask the doctor to write down how often and for how long you should take it.

CAN I FIND INFORMATION ABOUT MEDICAL TESTS ONLINE?

Yes—there is a lot of information on the Internet about medical tests. The National Library of Medicine's MedlinePlus website provides links to many trustworthy resources. Visit www.medlineplus.gov and enter "laboratory tests" in the search window at the top of the page. Then, select the link that applies to your situation. You can get information on preparing for lab tests, explanations of different tests, and tips on interpreting lab test results.

Make notes about any other special instructions. There may be foods or drinks you should avoid while you are taking the medicine. Or you may have to take the medicine with food or a whole glass of water. If you are taking other medications, make sure your doctor knows, so he or she can prevent harmful drug interactions.

Sometimes medicines affect older people differently than younger people. Let the doctor know if your medicine doesn't seem to be working or if it is causing problems. It is best not to stop taking the medicine on your own. If you want to stop taking your medicine, check with your doctor first.

If another doctor (for example, a specialist) prescribes a medication for you, call your primary doctor's office and leave a message letting him or her know. Also call to check with your doctor's office before taking any over-the-counter medications. You may find it helpful to keep a chart of all the medicines you take and when you take them.

The pharmacist is also a good source of information about your medicines. In addition to answering questions and helping you select over-the-counter medications, the pharmacist keeps records of all the prescriptions you get filled at that pharmacy. Because your pharmacist keeps these records, it is helpful to use the same store regularly. At your request, the pharmacist can fill your prescriptions in easy-to-open containers and may be able to provide large-print prescription labels.

WHAT ARE SIDE EFFECTS?

"My headache prescription always makes me sleepy." "Aunt Sarah's cough syrup caused a rash."

Unwanted or unexpected symptoms or feelings that happen when you take a medicine are called side effects.

Some side effects happen just when you start taking a medicine. Some happen only once in a while and you learn how to manage them. But other side effects may make you want to stop taking the medicine. Tell your doctor if this happens. He or she may be able to prescribe a different medicine or help you deal with these side effects in other ways.

Questions to ask about medications:

- What are the common side effects? What should I pay attention to?
- When will the medicine begin to work?
- What should I do if I miss a dose?
- Should I take it at meals or between meals? Do I need to drink a whole glass of water with it?

- Are there foods, drugs, or activities I should avoid while taking this medicine?
- Will I need a refill? How do I arrange that?

Understand your prescriptions — When the doctor writes you a prescription, it is important that you are able to read and understand the directions for taking the medication. Doctors and pharmacists often use abbreviations or terms that may not be familiar. Here is an explanation of some of the most common abbreviations you will see on the labels of your prescription medications:

p.r.n.	as needed	a.c.	before meals
q.d.	every day	p.c.	after meals
b.i.d.	twice a day	h.s.	at bedtime
t.i.d.	three times a day	p.o.	by mouth
q.i.d.	four times a day	ea.	each

If you have questions about your prescription or how you should take the medicine, ask your doctor or pharmacist. If you do not understand the directions, make sure you ask someone to explain them. It is important to take the medicine as directed by your doctor.

Keeping a record of the medications you take and the instructions for taking them can help you get the most benefit from them

Summary: Getting Information

- Learn about medical tests.
- Discuss your diagnosis and what you can expect.
- Find out about your medications.
- Understand how to take your prescriptions.

TIPS: HELPING YOU REMEMBER

No matter what your age, it's easy to forget a lot of what your doctor says. Even if you are comfortable talking with your doctor, you may not always understand what he or she says.

How Can I be Involved? Making Decisions with Your Doctor

Giving and getting information are two important steps in talking with your doctor. The third big step is making decisions about your care.

Ask about different treatments — You will benefit most from a treatment when you know what is happening and are involved in making decisions. Make sure you understand what your treatment involves and what it will or will not do. Have the doctor give you directions in writing and feel free to ask questions. For example: *"What are the pros and cons of having surgery at this stage?"* or *"Do I have any other choices?"*

If your doctor suggests a treatment that makes you uncomfortable, ask if there are other treatments that might work. If cost is a concern, ask the doctor if less expensive choices are available. The doctor can work with you to develop a treatment plan that meets your needs.

Here are some things to remember when deciding on a treatment:

- **Discuss choices.** There are different ways to manage many health conditions, especially chronic conditions like high blood pressure and cholesterol. Ask what your options are.
- **Discuss risks and benefits.** Once you know your options, ask about the pros and cons of each one. Find out what side effects might occur, how long the treatment would continue, and how likely it is that the treatment will work for you.
- **Consider your own values and circumstances.** When thinking about the pros and cons of a treatment, don't forget to consider its impact on your overall life. For instance, will one of the side effects interfere with a regular activity that means a lot to you? Is one treatment choice expensive and not covered by your insurance? Doctors need to know about these practical matters and can work with you to develop a treatment plan that meets your needs.

Ask about prevention — Doctors and other health professionals may suggest you change your diet, activity level, or other aspects of your life to help you deal with medical conditions. Research has shown that these changes, particularly an increase in exercise, have positive effects on overall health.

So, as your doctor gives you information, it's a good idea to check that you are following along. Ask about anything that does not seem clear. For instance, you might say: *"I want to make sure I understand. Could you explain that a little more?"* or *"I did not understand that word. What does it mean?"*

Another way to check is to repeat what you think the doctor means in your own words and ask, *"Is this correct?"* Here are some other ideas to help make sure you have all the information you need.

Take notes — Take along a notepad and pencil and write down the main points, or ask the doctor to write them down for you. If you can't write while the doctor is talking to you, make notes in the waiting room after the visit. Or, bring a tape recorder along, and (with the doctor's permission) record what is said. Recording is especially helpful if you want to share the details of the visit with others.

Get written or recorded materials — Ask if your doctor has any brochures, DVDs, CDs, cassettes, or videotapes about your health conditions or treatments. For example, if your doctor says that your blood pressure is high, he or she may give you brochures explaining what causes high blood pressure and what you can do about it. Ask the doctor to recommend other sources, such as websites, public libraries, nonprofit organizations, and government agencies that may have written or recorded information you can use.

Talk to other members of the health care team — Sometimes the doctor may want you to talk with other health professionals who can help you understand and carry out the decisions about how to manage your condition. Nurses, physician assistants, pharmacists, and occupational or physical therapists may be able to take more time with you than the doctor.

Call or email the doctor — If you are uncertain about the doctor's instructions after you get home, call the office. A nurse or other staff member can check with the doctor and call you back. You could ask whether the doctor, or other health professional you have talked to, has an email address you can use to send questions.

> ## TALKING ABOUT EXERCISE
>
> Exercise is often "just what the doctor ordered!" Exercise can:
>
> - Help you have more energy to do the things you want to do.
> - Help maintain and improve your physical strength and fitness.
> - Help improve mood and relieve depression.
> - Help manage and prevent diseases like heart disease, diabetes, some types of cancer, osteoporosis, and disabilities as people grow older.
> - Help improve your balance.
>
> Many doctors now recommend that older people try to make physical activity a part of everyday life. When you are making your list of things to talk about with your doctor, add exercise. Ask how exercise would benefit you, if there are any activities you should avoid, and whether your doctor can recommend any specific kinds of exercise.

Until recently, preventing disease in older people received little attention. But things are changing. We now know that it's never too late to stop smoking, improve your diet, or start exercising. Getting regular checkups and seeing other health professionals such as dentists and eye specialists helps promote good health. Even people who have chronic diseases, like arthritis or diabetes, can prevent further disability and, in some cases, control the progress of the disease.

If a certain disease or health condition runs in your family, ask your doctor if there are steps you can take to help prevent it. If you have a chronic condition, ask how you can manage it and if there are things you can do to prevent it from getting worse. If you want to discuss health and disease prevention with your doctor, say so when you make your next appointment. This lets the doctor plan to spend more time with you.

It is just as important to talk with your doctor about lifestyle changes as it is to talk about treatment. For example: *"I know that you've told me to eat more dairy products, but they really disagree with me. Is there something else I could eat instead?"* or *"Maybe an exercise class would help, but I have no way to get to the senior center. Is there something else you could suggest?"*

Just as with treatments, consider all the alternatives, look at pros and cons, and remember to take into account your own point of view. Tell your doctor if you feel his or her suggestions won't work for you and explain why. Keep talking with your doctor to come up with a plan that works.

SUMMARY: MAKING DECISIONS WITH YOUR DOCTOR

Ask about different treatments:

- Are there any risks associated with the treatment?
- How soon should treatment start? How long will it last?
- Are there other treatments available?
- How much will the treatment cost? Will my insurance cover it?

Ask about prevention:

- Is there any way to prevent a condition that runs in my family—before it affects me?
- Are there ways to keep my condition from getting worse?
- How will making a change in my habits help me?
- Are there any risks in making this change?
- Are there support groups or community services that might help me?

TIPS: EVALUATING HEALTH INFORMATION ON THE INTERNET

Many people search the Internet to find information about medical problems and health issues. However, not all health information on the web is of equal quality. How do you find websites that are accurate and reliable? The following questions may be useful to consider when you look at a health-related website.

- Who is responsible for the content? Is it a government agency, national nonprofit organization, or professional association? An individual? A commercial organization?

- If you are reading a particular article, what are the author's credentials? Is the author affiliated with any major medical institutions?
- Who reviews the material? Is there a medical advisory board that reads the medical content before it is made available to the public?
- Are sources cited for the statistical information? For example, it's easy enough to say "4 out of 5 doctors agree..." but where did that statistic come from?
- Is the purpose and goal of the sponsoring organization clearly stated?
- Is there a way to contact the sponsor for more information or to verify information presented?
- Is the site supported by public funds or donations? If it includes advertisements, are they separate from content?
- Because health information gets outdated so quickly, does the website post the source and date for the information?
- If you have to register, is it clear how your personal information will be used? Does the site have a clear privacy policy?
- Is the website trying to sell you something?

Don't forget to talk with your doctor about what you've learned online.

ASKING MORE QUESTIONS: TALKING TO DOCTORS IN SPECIAL SITUATIONS

Your doctor may send you to a specialist for further evaluation, or you may request to see a specialist yourself. It's likely that your insurance plan will require you to have a referral from your primary doctor.

A visit to the specialist may be short. Often, the specialist already has seen your medical records or test results and is familiar with your case. If you are unclear about what the specialist tells you, ask questions.

For example, if the specialist says that you have a medical condition that you aren't familiar with, you may want to say something like: *"I don't know very much about that condition. Could you explain what it is and how it might affect me?"* or *"I've heard that is a painful problem. What can be done to prevent or manage the pain?"*

You also may ask for written materials to read, or you can call your primary doctor to clarify anything you haven't understood.

Ask the specialist to send information about any further diagnosis or treatment to your primary doctor. This allows your primary doctor to keep track of your medical care. You also should let your primary doctor know at your next visit how well any treatments or medications the specialist recommended are working.

Questions to ask your specialist:

- What is your diagnosis?
- What treatment do you recommend? How soon do I need to begin the new treatment?
- Will you discuss my care with my primary doctor?

If you need to have surgery — In some cases, surgery may be the best treatment for your condition. If so, your doctor will refer you to a surgeon. Knowing more about the operation will help you make an informed decision about how to proceed. It also will help you get ready for the surgery, which makes for a better recovery.

Ask the surgeon to explain what will be done during the operation and what reading material, videotapes, or websites you can look at before the operation.

Find out if you will have to stay overnight in the hospital or if the surgery can be done on an outpatient basis. Will you need someone to drive you home? Minor surgeries that don't require an overnight stay can sometimes be done at medical centers called ambulatory surgical centers.

Questions to ask your surgeon:

- What is the success rate of the operation? How many of these operations have you done successfully?
- What problems occur with this surgery? What kind of pain or discomfort can I expect?
- What kind of anesthesia will I have? Are there any risks associated with it for older people?

- Will I have to stay in the hospital overnight? How long is recovery expected to take? What does it involve? When can I get back to my normal routine?

If you are hospitalized — If you have to go to the hospital, some extra guidelines may help you. First, most hospitals have a daily schedule. Knowing the hospital routine can make your stay more comfortable. Find out how much choice you have about your daily routine and express any preferences you have about your schedule. Doctors generally visit patients during specific times each day. Find out when the doctor is likely to visit so you can have your questions ready.

In the hospital, your primary doctor and various medical specialists, as well as nurses and other health professionals, may examine you. If you are in a teaching hospital, doctors-in-training known as medical students, interns, residents, or fellows, also may examine you. Many of these doctors-in-training already have a lot of knowledge and experience. They may be able to take more time to talk with you than other staff. Nurses also can be an important source of information, especially since you will see them often.

Questions to ask medical staff in the hospital:

- How long can I expect to be in the hospital?
- When will I see my doctor? What doctors and health professionals will I see?
- What is the daily routine in this part of the hospital?

If you go to the emergency room — A visit to the emergency room can be stressful. It may go more smoothly if you can take along the following items:

- Your health insurance card or policy number.
- A list of your medications.
- A list of your medical problems.
- The names and phone numbers of your doctor and one or two family members or close friends.

Some people find it helpful to keep this information on a card in their wallet or purse at all times.

> ## SEEKING A SECOND OPINION
>
> When surgery is recommended, patients often seek a second opinion. Hearing the views of two different doctors can help you decide what's best for you. In fact, your insurance plan may require it. Doctors are used to this practice, and most will not be insulted by your request for a second opinion. Your doctor may even be able to suggest other doctors who can review your case.
>
> Always remember to check with your insurance provider in advance to find out whether a second opinion is covered under your policy, if there are restrictions to which doctors you can see, and if you need a referral form from your primary doctor.

Depending on the problem, you may have a long wait in the emergency room. Consider taking things to make the wait more comfortable, such as something to read or a sweater in case the room is cold.

While in the emergency room, ask questions if you don't understand tests or procedures that are being done. Before leaving, make sure you understand what the doctor told you or ask for written instructions. For example, if you have bandages that need changing, be sure you understand how and when it should be done. Tell your primary doctor as soon as possible about your visit to the emergency room.

Questions to ask medical staff in the emergency room:

- Will you talk to my primary doctor about my care?
- Do I need to arrange any further care?
- May I get instructions for further care in writing?
- Is there someone here who speaks my language and can explain the instructions?

Summary: Talking to Doctors in Special Situations

- Ask questions if you are unclear.

- Try to write down as much information as possible.
- Tell your primary care doctor if you see a specialist, need surgery, or have gone to the emergency room.

TO CHANGE THE SUBJECT: PRACTICAL MATTERS

It helps the doctor—and you—if he or she knows about the non-medical parts of your life. Where you live, how you get around, what activities are important to you: these are all things that can make a difference in decisions about your health care. The following are some examples of practical matters you might want to discuss with your doctor. For more information and resources on these topics, see the section on additional resources included at the end of this booklet.

Planning for care in the event of a serious illness — You may have some concerns or wishes about your care if you become seriously ill. If you have questions about what choices you have, ask your doctor. You can specify your desires through documents called advance directives, such as a living will or health care proxy. One way to bring up the subject is to say: *"I'm worried about what would happen in the hospital if I were very sick and not likely to get better. Can you tell me what generally happens in that case?"*

In general, the best time to talk with your doctor about these issues is when you are still relatively healthy. If you are admitted to the hospital or a nursing home, a nurse or other staff member may ask if you have any advance directives.

Driving — Driving is an important part of everyday life for many people and making the decision to stop driving can be very difficult. Tell your doctor if you or people close to you are concerned about your driving and why. He or she can go over your medical conditions and medications to see if there are treatable problems that may be contributing to driving difficulties. Vision and memory tests are important. The doctor also may be able to suggest a driver's education refresher class designed for older drivers.

Moving to assisted living — Another hard decision that many older people face is whether or not to move to a place where they can have more help—often an assisted living facility. If you are considering such a move, your doctor can help you weigh the pros and cons based on your health and other circumstances. He or she may be able to refer you to a social worker or a local agency that can help in finding an assisted living facility.

Paying for medications — Don't hesitate to ask the doctor about the cost of your medications. If they are too expensive for you, the doctor may be able to suggest less expensive alternatives. If the doctor does not know the cost, ask the pharmacist before filling the prescription. Then call your doctor and ask if there is a generic or other less expensive choice. You could say, for instance: *"It turns out that this medicine is too expensive for me. Is there another one or a generic drug that would cost less?"*

Your doctor may also be able to refer you to a medical assistance program that can help with drug costs.

Summary: Practical Matters

- Don't hesitate to bring up concerns, even if they don't seem directly related to a medical condition.
- You and your doctor can make better decisions together if the doctor knows about your troubling non-medical concerns.
- If the doctor can't help solve your non-medical problems, he or she may be able to refer you to other resources that can help.

TIPS: ADVANCE DIRECTIVES

Advance directives are written instructions letting others know the type of care you want if you are seriously ill or dying. There are two main kinds:

Living wills — A living will records your end-of-life wishes for medical treatment in case you are no longer able to speak for yourself. Living wills typically refer only to life- prolonging treatment when you are close to death.

Health care proxies — A health care proxy is named through a "durable power of attorney for health care." Sometimes this person may be referred to as a representative, surrogate, agent, or attorney-in-fact.

> A health care proxy is helpful if you do not want to be specific about your end-of-life treatment—you would rather let the health care proxy evaluate each situation or treatment option independently. This type of advance directive is also important if you want your health care proxy to be someone who is not a legal member of your family.
>
> Make sure your doctor and family understand your advance directives and your views about end-of-life care. That will help them make the decisions you would want. Sometimes people change their mind as they get older or after they become ill. Review the choices in your advance care directives from time to time and make changes as needed.
>
> Advance care directives are legally valid everywhere in the United States, but laws concerning them vary from state to state. Forms approved for the state you live in are available from many different health care organizations and institutions. Make sure that the form you choose is legal in your home state and any other state that you may live in for part of the year.

CAN I REALLY TALK ABOUT THAT? DISCUSSING SENSITIVE SUBJECTS

Much of the communication between doctor and patient is personal. To have a good partnership with your doctor, it is important to talk about sensitive subjects, like sex or memory problems, even if you are embarrassed or uncomfortable. Most doctors are used to talking about personal matters and will try to ease your discomfort. Keep in mind that these topics concern many older people. You might find that using booklets from these organizations can help you bring up sensitive subjects when talking with your doctor.

It is important to understand that problems with memory, depression, sexual function, and incontinence are not necessarily normal parts of aging. A good doctor will take your concerns about these topics seriously and not brush them off as being "normal." If you think your doctor isn't taking your concerns seriously, talk to him or her about your feelings or consider looking for a new doctor.

Alcohol — Anyone at any age can have a drinking problem. Alcohol can have a greater effect as a person grows older because the aging process affects how the body handles alcohol. Someone whose drinking habits haven't changed may find over time that he or she has a problem. People can also develop a drinking problem later in life due to major life changes like the death of loved ones. In fact, depression in older adults often goes along with alcohol misuse. Talk to your doctor if you think you may be developing a drinking problem. You could say: *"Lately I've been wanting to have a drink earlier and earlier in the afternoon and I find it's getting harder to stop after just one or two. What kind of treatments could help with this?"*

Falling and fear of falling — A fall can be a serious event, often leading to injury and loss of independence, at least for a while. For this reason, many older people develop a fear of falling. Studies show that fear of falling can keep people from going about their normal activities, and as a result they may become frailer, which actually increases their risk of falling again. If fear of falling is affecting your day-to-day life, let your doctor know. He or she may be able to recommend some things to do to reduce your chances of falling. Exercises can help you improve your balance and strengthen your muscles, at any age.

Feeling unhappy with your doctor — Misunderstandings can come up in any relationship, including between a patient and doctor or the doctor's staff. If you feel uncomfortable with something your doctor or his or her staff has said or done, be direct. For example, if the doctor does not return your telephone calls, you may want to say something like this: *"I realize that you care for a lot of patients and are very busy, but I feel frustrated when I have to wait for days for you to return my call. Is there a way we can work together to improve this?"*

Being honest is much better for your health than avoiding the doctor. If you have a long-standing relationship with your doctor, working out the problem may be more useful than looking for a new doctor.

Grief, mourning, and depression — As people grow older, they may lose significant people in their lives, including spouses and cherished friends. Or they may have to move away from home or give up favorite activities. A doctor who knows about your losses is better able to understand how you are feeling. He or she can make suggestions that may be helpful to you.

Although it is normal to mourn when you have a loss, later life does not have to be a time of ongoing sadness. If you feel sad all the time or for more than a few weeks, let your doctor know. Also tell your doctor about symptoms such as lack of energy, poor appetite, trouble sleeping, or little interest in life. These could be signs of depression, which is a medical condition.

> ## FREE INFORMATION
>
> If you are worried about memory problems and Alzheimer's disease, you can contact the NIA-funded Alzheimer's Disease Education and Referral Center (ADEAR)— a comprehensive source of information. ADEAR staff can:
>
> - Answer specific questions about Alzheimer's disease.
> - Send free publications.
> - Refer callers to local resources.
> - Provide information about clinical trials.
> - Help you find materials about specific issues.
>
> Call toll-free 1-800-438-4380 or visit the ADEAR website at www.nia.nih.gov/Alzheimers.

Depression may be common, especially when people experience losses, but it is also treatable. It should not be considered "normal" at any age. Let your doctor know about your feelings and ask about treatment.

HIV/AIDS — The death of a spouse, divorce, or separation can lead some older people to find themselves dating again and possibly having sex with a new partner. It's a good idea to talk to your doctor about how safe sex can reduce your risk of sexually transmitted diseases such as HIV/AIDS. It's important to practice safe sex, no matter what your age.

Incontinence — Older people sometimes have problems controlling their bladder. This is called urinary incontinence and it can often be treated. Depending on the type of incontinence you have, the doctor may recommend exercises, suggest helpful ways to change your habits, prescribe useful medications, or advise surgery. If you have trouble controlling your bladder or bowels, it is important to let the doctor know. To bring up the topic, you could say something like: *"Since my last visit there have been several times that I couldn't control my bladder."*

Memory problems — Many older people worry about their ability to think and remember. For most older adults, thinking and memory remain relatively intact in later years. However, if you or your family notice that you are having problems remembering recent events or thinking clearly, let your doctor know. Be specific about the changes you've noticed; for example, you could say: *"I've always been able to balance my checkbook without any problems, but lately I'm very confused."* Your doctor will probably want you to have a thorough checkup to see what might be causing your symptoms. In many cases, memory problems are caused by conditions such as depression or infection, or they may be a side effect of medication. Sometimes the problem is a type of dementia, such as Alzheimer's disease. With a careful history, physical exam, medical tests, and tests of memory and problem solving, specialists can diagnose Alzheimer's with a high degree of accuracy. Determining the cause of memory problems is important to help the doctor, patient, and family choose the best plan of care. Although there is no cure for Alzheimer's, medicines can help for a while, especially in the early stages of the disease. Medications also can ease serious behavioral symptoms such as agitation, anxiety, and depression. Support groups and education are important and can help patients and caregivers.

Problems with family — Even strong and loving families can have problems, especially under the stress of illness. Although family problems can be painful to discuss, talking about them can help your doctor help you. Your doctor may be able to suggest steps to improve the situation for you and other family members.

If you feel that a family member or caregiver is taking advantage of you or mistreating you, let your doctor know. Some older people are subjected to abuse by family members or others. Abuse can be physical, verbal, psychological, or even financial in nature. Your doctor may be able to provide resources or referrals to other services that can help if you are being mistreated.

Sexuality — Most health professionals now understand that sexuality remains important in later life. If you are not satisfied with your sex life, don't just assume it's due to your age. In addition to talking about age-related changes, you can ask your doctor about the effects of an illness or a disability on sexual function. Also, ask your doctor about the influence medications or surgery may have on your sex life. If you aren't sure how to bring the topic up, try saying: *"I have a personal question I would like to ask you..."* or *"I *understand that this condition or medication can affect my body in many ways. Will it affect my sex life at all?"*

Summary: Discussing Sensitive Subjects

- Don't hesitate to discuss sensitive subjects with your doctor.
- Use brochures or booklets as props to introduce topics you may feel awkward discussing.
- If you feel the doctor doesn't take your concerns seriously, it might be time to think about changing doctors.

WHO ELSE WILL HELP? INVOLVING YOUR FAMILY AND FRIENDS

It can be helpful to take a family member or friend with you when you go to the doctor's office. You may feel more confident if someone else is with you. Also, a relative or friend can help remind you about things you planned to tell or ask the doctor. He or she also can help you remember what the doctor says.

Don't let your companion take too strong a role. The visit is between you and the doctor. You may want some time alone with the doctor to discuss personal matters. If you are alone with the doctor during or right after the physical exam, this might be a good time to raise private concerns. Or, you could ask your family member or friend to stay in the waiting room for part of the appointment. For best results, let your companion know in advance how he or she can be most helpful.

If a relative or friend helps with your care at home, bringing that person along when you visit the doctor may be useful. In addition to the questions you have, your caregiver may have concerns he or she wants to discuss with the doctor. Some things caregivers may find especially helpful to discuss are: what to expect in the future, sources of information and support, community services, and ways they can maintain their own well-being.

Even if a family member or friend can't go with you to your appointment, he or she can still help. For example, the person can serve as your sounding board, helping you practice what you want to say to the doctor before the visit.

And after the visit, talking about what the doctor said can remind you of the important points and help you come up with questions to ask next time.

ADDITIONAL RESOURCES: FOR MORE INFORMATION

You can make the most of your time with your doctor by being informed. This often includes drawing on other sources of health information such as the Internet, home medical guides, books and articles available at libraries, national organizations or associations, other institutes within the National Institutes of Health, and self-help groups.

NIA has free information in English and Spanish. Call the NIA Information Center at 1-800-222-2225 or TTY at 1-800-222-4225 to order publications or request a publications catalog. Publications can be ordered online by visiting www.nia.nih.gov/HealthInformation; you can also sign up for email alerts about new NIA publications at this website. Spanish-language publications are also available at www.nia.nih.gov/Espanol. Publications from NIA are available in bulk—for example, you may want to encourage your doctor to order copies of this publication for his or her office.

For free fact sheets and other publications about Alzheimer's disease, contact the NIA's Alzheimer's Disease Education and Referral (ADEAR) Center at 1-800-438-4380. The ADEAR Center website is www.nia.nih.gov/Alzheimers.

Good health care depends on good communication with your doctor and other health care professionals. Let the ideas in this booklet help you take a more active role in your health care. The organizations on the next pages are a sampling of other resources that may also be useful.

NIHSeniorHealth.gov

The NIA and the National Library of Medicine, both part of the National Institutes of Health, have developed a website designed specifically for older people. The website features a wide variety of popular health topics presented in a simple-to- use, easy-to-read format. It also has short videos and a "talking web" feature that reads the text to you. Visit this website at www.nihseniorhealth.gov.

General Resources

NIA Information Center
P.O. Box 8057
Gaithersburg, MD 20898-8057
1-800-222-2225
1-800-222-4225 (TTY)
www.nia.nih.gov/HealthInformation
www.nihseniorhealth.gov
www.nia.nih.gov/Espanol

National Institutes of Health
9000 Rockville Pike
Bethesda, MD 20892
1-301-496-4000
1-301-402-9612 (TTY)
www.nih.gov

MedlinePlus
c/o National Library of Medicine
8600 Rockville Pike
Bethesda, MD 20894
1-888-FIND-NLM (1-888-346-3656)
1-800-735-2258 (TDD)
www.medlineplus.gov

Medicare
Centers for Medicare and Medicaid Services
7500 Security Boulevard
Baltimore, MD 21244-1850
1-800-MEDICARE (1-800-633-4227)
1-877-486-2048 (TTY)
www.medicare.gov

AARP (formerly the American Association of Retired Persons)
601 E Street, NW Washington, DC 20049
1-888-OUR-AARP (1-888-687-2277)

1-877-434-7598 (TTY)
www.aarp.org

Advance Directives

Patient Education Forum: Advance Directives
The American Geriatrics Society
The Empire State Building
350 Fifth Avenue, Suite 801
New York, NY 10118
1-800-563-4916
www.healthinaging.org/public_ education/pef/advance_directives.php

Alcohol

National Institute on Alcohol Abuse and Alcoholism
5635 Fishers Lane, MSC 9304
Bethesda, MD 20892-9304
1-301-443-3860
www.niaaa.nih.gov

Substance Abuse and Mental Health Services Administration
P.O. Box 2345
Rockville, MD 20847-2345
1-877-SAMHSA-7 (1-877-726-4727)
1-800-487-4889 (TTY)
www.samhsa.gov

Assisted Living

Assisted Living Federation of America
1650 King Street, Suite 602
Alexandria, VA 22314-2747
1-703-894-1805
www.alfa.org

National Center for Assisted Living
1201 L Street, NW
Washington, DC 20005
1-202-842-4444
www.ncal.org

Housing Choices
AARP
601 E Street, NW
Washington, DC 20049
1-888-OUR-AARP (1-888-687-2277)
1-877-434-7598 (TTY)
www.aarp.org/home-garden/housing/

Care in the Event of a Terminal Illness

National Hospice and Palliative Care Organization
1731 King Street, Suite 100
Alexandria, VA 22314
1-800-658-8898
1-877-658-8896 (multilingual)
www.nhpco.org

Driving

SeniorDrivers.org
AAA Foundation for Traffic Safety
Administrative Office
607 14th Street, NW, Suite 201
Washington, DC 20005-2000
1-202-638-5944
www.seniordrivers.org

AARP Driver Safety Program
601 E Street, NW
Washington, DC 20049
1-888-OUR-AARP (1-888-687-2277)

1-877-434-7598 (TTY)
www.aarp.org/home-garden/transportation/driver_safety/

Patient Education Forum: Safe Driving for Seniors
The American Geriatrics Society
The Empire State Building
350 Fifth Avenue, Suite 801
New York, NY 10118
1-800-563-4916
www.healthinaging.org/public_education/pef/safe_driving_for_seniors.php

Exercise

American College of Sports Medicine
P.O. Box 1440
Indianapolis, IN 46206-1440
1-317-637-9200
www.acsm.org

Centers for Disease Control and Prevention
1600 Clifton Road
Atlanta, GA 30333
1-800-CDC-INFO (1-800-232-4636)
1-888-232-6348 (TTY)
www.cdc.gov

The President's Council on Physical Fitness and Sports
Department W
Tower Building, Suite 560
1101 Wootton Parkway
Rockville, MD 20852
1-240-276-9567
www.fitness.gov

Grief, Mourning, and Depression

>National Institute of Mental Health
>6001 Executive Boulevard
>Room 8184, MSC 9663
>Bethesda, MD 20892-9663
>1-866-615-6464
>1-866-415-8051 (TTY)
>www.nimh.nih.gov

HIV/AIDS

>National Association on HIV Over Fifty
>23 Miner Street
>Ground Level
>Boston, MA 02215-3319
>1-617-233-7107
>www.hivoverfifty.org

Incontinence

>National Association for Continence
>P.O. Box 1019
>Charleston, SC 29402-1019
>1-800-BLADDER (1-800-252-3337)
>www.nafc.org

>The Simon Foundation for Continence
>P.O. Box 815
>Wilmette, IL 60091
>1-800-23-SIMON (1-800-237-4666)
>www.simonfoundation.org

Medication

Center for Drug Evaluation and Research
U.S. Food and Drug Administration
10903 New Hampshire Avenue
Silver Spring, MD 20993
1-888-INFO-FDA (1-888-463-6332)
www.fda.gov/AboutFDA/CentersOffices/CDER/default.htm

Medicare
Centers for Medicare and Medicaid Services
7500 Security Boulevard
Baltimore, MD 21244-1850
1-800-MEDICARE (1-800-633-4227)
1-877-486-2048 (TTY)
www.medicare.gov

Memory Problems

Alzheimer's Disease Education and Referral Center
P.O. Box 8250
Silver Spring, MD 20907
1-800-438-4380
www.nia.nih.gov/Alzheimers

Alzheimer's Association
225 North Michigan Avenue, Floor 17
Chicago, IL 60601-7633
1-800-272-3900
1-866-403-3073 (TDD)
www.alz.org

Problems with Family/Caregiving

Children of Aging Parents
P.O. Box 167
Richboro, PA 18954-0167

1-800-227-7294
www.caps4caregivers.org

Eldercare Locator Service
1-800-677-1116 (bilingual)
www.eldercare.gov

National Center on Elder Abuse
U.S. Administration on Aging
c/o University of Delaware
297 Graham Hall
Newark, DE 19716
1-302-831-3525
www.ncea.aoa.gov

Sexuality

Sexuality Information and Education Council of the United States
1706 R Street, NW
Washington, DC 20009
1-202-265-2405
www.siecus.org

INDEX

A

abuse, 25, 26, 90
access, 16, 40, 42
activity level, 78
AD, 48, 49, 51
adults, 5, 9, 19, 20, 25, 29, 31, 32, 35, 46, 48, 55, 88, 90
advertisements, 81
age, viii, 4, 10, 20, 21, 22, 24, 31, 32, 33, 34, 62, 66, 76, 87, 88, 89, 90
agencies, 51, 77
aging process, 87
AIDS, 57, 89
alcohol use, 16
alternative medicine, 42
alternative treatments, 15, 65
aneurysm, 73
anger, 10, 39
anticholinergic, 50
anxiety, 49, 53, 90
appetite, 68, 89
appointments, 38, 39, 41, 48, 54, 66
arthritis, 79
assessment, 50
attitudes, 15, 16
authority, 47

B

baby boomers, 4, 5, 32
background information, 52
background noise, 10
barriers, 5
behavioral change, 48
benefits, vii, 1, 6, 18, 20, 59, 78
biopsy, 39
blame, 39
blood, 73, 77
blood pressure, 77
breast cancer, 18

C

calcium, 20
campaigns, 29
cancer, 11, 79
candidates, 65
car accidents, 25
cardiovascular disease, 18
caregivers, 3, 14, 25, 26, 35, 36, 37, 38, 45, 46, 47, 48, 50, 51, 53, 54, 58, 90, 91
caregiving, 28, 46
CAT scan, 9
CDC, 19, 96
Census, 42
certification, 32, 64

challenges, 32, 35, 47, 48, 53
Chicago, 25, 27, 50, 55, 98
children, 3, 40, 47, 69
cholesterol, 78
chronic diseases, 19, 79
classes, 19, 24
clinical trials, 40, 51, 89
cognition, 48, 49
cognitive abilities, 26
cognitive capacity, 52
cognitive function, 48, 49, 53
cognitive impairment, 47, 48, 49, 50, 52, 53
colon, 18, 39
colon cancer, 18, 39
colorectal cancer, 73
commercial, 80
communication, vii, viii, 1, 2, 4, 5, 6, 9, 11, 46, 49, 54, 61, 62, 64, 66, 69, 73, 87, 92
communication skills, vii, 1, 2, 9, 64
communication strategies, 9
community, 6, 19, 20, 28, 34, 35, 46, 50, 51, 59, 68, 69, 70, 80, 91
community service, 51, 80, 91
community-based services, 46
complications, 15
conference, 53, 54
confidentiality, 22
conflict, 41
consent, 37, 53, 54
consulting, 4
containers, 75
conversations, 29, 39
cooking, 16, 48
cooperation, 7, 54
cost, 37, 63, 66, 73, 78, 80, 86
cough, 34, 75
counseling, 28, 54
covering, 49
credentials, 63, 81
cues, 26, 30
cultural differences, 44
culture, 42
cure, 33, 34, 90
curricula, 9

D

daily living, 16, 17
dance, 18
database, 51
defibrillator, 25
dementia, 11, 18, 90
denial, 39
Department of Agriculture, 19
depression, 20, 22, 29, 53, 68, 79, 87, 88, 89, 90
depressive symptoms, 6
depth, 57
despair, 39
detection, 33
diabetes, 18, 79
diagnosis, vii, 2, 4, 39, 48, 49, 50, 51, 53, 68, 74, 76, 82
diet, 37, 72, 78, 79
directives, 15, 22, 23, 24, 27, 34, 39, 49, 85, 86, 87, 94
disability, 4, 79, 90
discomfort, 2, 4, 26, 82, 87
diseases, 15, 33, 79
disorder, 51, 70
distress, 31
dizziness, 25
doctors, vii, 4, 7, 15, 25, 29, 44, 62, 63, 64, 65, 67, 68, 70, 72, 73, 79, 81, 83, 84, 87, 91
donations, 81
dosage, 45
drawing, 92
drug abuse, 32
drug interaction, 75
drugs, 32, 33, 37, 41, 71, 76

E

education, 16, 32, 43, 47, 51, 55, 64, 85, 90, 94, 96
educational materials, 34
educational programs, 55
educators, 56

emergency, 13, 66, 68, 69, 83, 84, 85
emotional distress, 39
empathy, 8
emphysema, 35, 40
empirical studies, 5
encouragement, 18, 36, 47, 50
endurance, 19, 20
energy, 18, 20, 29, 35, 68, 79, 89
equipment, 10, 17
ethics, 39
ethnic background, 41
etiquette, 5
everyday life, 79, 85
evidence, 70
exercise, 17, 18, 19, 21, 37, 54, 78, 79
expertise, 64
extra help, 29

F

families, vii, 2, 7, 24, 32, 34, 46, 50, 51, 58, 90
family history, 12, 13, 15, 17, 26, 49
family members, 5, 14, 15, 16, 23, 26, 35, 39, 42, 44, 47, 49, 53, 54, 83, 90
FDA, 98
fear, 4, 13, 26, 48, 88
fears, 5, 40
Federal funds, 42
feelings, 49, 62, 72, 75, 87, 89
fever, 70
financial, 16, 27, 28, 47, 49, 51, 90
fitness, 19, 79, 96
flexibility, 19, 20
flu shot, 67
food, 20, 21, 41, 42, 73, 74
Food and Drug Administration, 98
formal language, 6
foundations, 44
framing, 31
funding, 44
funds, 30, 46, 55, 81

G

Georgia, 19
gestures, 42
glasses, 67
glaucoma, 73
good communication, vii, viii, 1, 11, 61, 62, 73, 92
GSA, 56
guidance, 25, 53
guidelines, 13, 51, 83
guilt, 39

H

headache, 75
healing, 1
health care, vii, viii, 2, 3, 4, 5, 12, 13, 16, 17, 22, 23, 27, 28, 31, 32, 35, 39, 40, 41, 42, 43, 45, 47, 48, 51, 53, 61, 62, 63, 65, 70, 77, 85, 86, 87, 92
health care costs, 27, 28
health care professionals, 2, 3, 13, 32, 51, 92
health care system, 35, 45
health condition, viii, 35, 62, 77, 78, 79
health information, 5, 51, 80, 81, 92
health insurance, 83
health problems, 6, 29, 37, 48
health services, 28
hearing impairment, 10
hearing loss, 10
heart disease, 3, 79
high blood pressure, 77, 78
history, 2, 12, 13, 16, 39, 50, 70, 90
HIV, 57, 89, 97
HIV/AIDS, 89, 97
homes, 3
hospice, 27
House, 17
housing, 95
husband, 31
hypertension, 18, 73

I

ID, 15
identity, 24
immigrants, 42
impairments, 2
income, 28
independence, 5, 20, 21, 22, 24, 35, 88
individuals, 3, 45
infection, 34, 90
informed consent, 49
injections, 47
injuries, 18, 25
injury, 88
insanity, 11
institutions, 81, 87
internists, 15, 62
intimacy, 30
investment, 2, 13, 16
issues, vii, 2, 4, 11, 15, 22, 26, 29, 43, 45, 46, 50, 54, 56, 80, 85, 89

K

kerosene, 13
kidney, 33

L

laboratory tests, 50, 74
language barrier, 68
languages, 68
later life, 88, 90
laws, 25, 87
laxatives, 71
lead, viii, 2, 6, 7, 15, 25, 61, 89
learning, 2, 16, 35, 65
level of education, 50
life changes, 88
life expectancy, 3
lifestyle changes, 18, 36, 37, 79
lifetime, 32
light, 11
literacy, 11, 12

living arrangements, 16, 17
loneliness, 6
longevity, 3
love, 6
lung disease, 13

M

majority, 30
malpractice suits, vii, 1
man, 48, 54, 62
management, vii, 1, 27, 33, 34, 35
marriage, 30
materials, 11, 12, 19, 20, 22, 23, 43, 44, 51, 55, 77, 82, 89
matter, 5, 62, 63, 66, 76, 89
Medicaid, 29, 44, 93, 98
medical, vii, viii, 4, 5, 6, 8, 9, 12, 13, 14, 15, 16, 23, 26, 27, 33, 35, 36, 39, 40, 42, 44, 45, 47, 49, 61, 62, 63, 64, 65, 67, 68, 70, 71, 73, 74, 76, 78, 80, 81, 82, 83, 84, 85, 86, 89, 90, 92
medical assistance, 86
medical care, 4, 5, 14, 82
medical expertise, 64
medical history, 13, 14, 49, 65, 70
medical students, 9, 83
Medicare, 27, 28, 29, 42, 64, 66, 93, 98
medication, 15, 17, 22, 28, 30, 33, 34, 37, 41, 45, 54, 69, 75, 76, 90, 91
medicine, 33, 42, 44, 64, 73, 74, 75, 76, 86
memory, 2, 7, 22, 48, 49, 51, 85, 87, 89, 90
memory loss, 2, 22, 48
mental disorder, 30
mental health, 29, 30, 39, 54
Miami, 20
misconceptions, 36
misuse, 15, 88
models, 36
modifications, 53
motivation, 18
muscles, 88
music, 49

Index

N

National Institute of Mental Health, 30, 97
National Institutes of Health, 2, 3, 30, 34, 43, 59, 92, 93
neglect, 25, 58
neon, 23
neurologist, 50, 51, 53
New England, 9
nonprofit organizations, 77
nurses, vii, viii, 2, 3, 25, 61, 83
nursing, 3, 15, 28, 29, 31, 58, 85
nursing home, 3, 15, 28, 29, 31, 58, 85
nutrients, 21
nutrition, 17, 19, 20, 21

O

obesity, 18
obstacles, 37
oil, 17
old age, 2, 3, 4
older patients, vii, viii, 1, 2, 4, 5, 6, 7, 9, 11, 12, 13, 15, 18, 21, 22, 25, 29, 35, 37, 41, 49, 54, 55, 56, 62, 65
operations, 70, 82
opportunities, 8, 26
osteoarthritis, 18
osteoporosis, 18, 54, 79
outpatient, 52, 82
oxygen, 13, 35

P

pain, 2, 15, 18, 27, 41, 70, 81, 82
parents, 17, 32
participants, 5
patient care, 55
patient- doctor relationship, viii, 61
permission, 70, 77
personal history, 39
pharmaceutical, 28
pharmacists, vii, viii, 61, 76, 77
physical activity, 17, 18, 19, 21, 79

physical therapist, 77
physicians, 2, 3, 5, 9, 11, 25, 27, 38
playing, 6, 49
police, 58
policy, 81, 83, 84
policymakers, 56
population, 42
prescription drugs, 67
President, 96
prevention, 33, 78, 79, 80
problem solving, 37, 90
professionals, 2, 25, 30, 46, 55, 63, 77, 78, 79, 83, 90
profit, 56
prognosis, 39, 41
public education, 55
public health, 32
public policy, 55

Q

qualifications, 64
quality of life, 18, 35, 53
questioning, 8

R

race, 66
Ramadan, 42
rash, 75
reaction time, 25
reactions, 39, 71
reading, 10, 11, 12, 13, 24, 81, 82
recommendations, 16, 54
recovery, 82, 83
reinforcement, 36
relatives, 15, 37, 63
religion, 66
requirements, 28
researchers, 3, 40, 56
resources, 19, 21, 22, 24, 28, 34, 35, 43, 44, 45, 46, 51, 53, 54, 55, 58, 59, 64, 68, 74, 85, 86, 89, 90, 92
response, 30

restrictions, 84
rewards, 8
risk(s), 17, 18, 31, 53, 78, 80, 82, 88, 89
rules, 42

S

sadness, 39, 88
safety, 16, 22, 24, 48, 50, 96
SAMHSA, 94
school, 9, 64
science, 55
sensory impairments, 9
services, 4, 20, 21, 28, 29, 34, 42, 44, 46, 50, 53, 58, 63, 90
sex, 30, 31, 66, 71, 87, 89, 90
sexual health, 31
sexuality, 22, 30, 31, 68, 69, 90
sexually transmitted diseases, 89
shock, 39
shortness of breath, 35
showing, 16
side effects, 33, 37, 71, 73, 75, 78
signs, 25, 29, 47, 89
smoking, 35, 72, 79
social services, 52
society, 32, 64
specialists, 62, 63, 79, 83, 90
spending, 49
spirituality, 31, 32
Spring, 51, 58, 98
staff members, 42
state, 87
stereotypes, 4
stigma, 29
stomach, 41, 73
stress, 7, 9, 16, 18, 26, 47, 50, 53, 90
stress test, 9
stroke, 18, 35
structure, 13, 15
style, 5
substance abuse, 32, 33
success rate, 82
suicide, 29
support services, 53

symptoms, 4, 5, 17, 25, 29, 37, 38, 49, 53, 68, 69, 70, 71, 72, 74, 75, 88, 90

T

TDD, 93, 98
team members, 36, 37
techniques, vii, 1, 2, 13, 21, 22, 34, 48, 54
teeth, 20
telephone, 49, 65, 88
testing, 49, 52
thoughts, 16, 65
time constraints, 2
tobacco, 16
traditions, 42
training, vii, 1, 2, 20, 34, 64, 83
transport, 59
transportation, 16, 17, 22, 25, 47, 96
treatment, vii, viii, 1, 2, 4, 7, 8, 12, 16, 17, 25, 27, 31, 32, 33, 34, 35, 36, 37, 38, 40, 41, 42, 45, 50, 61, 67, 71, 72, 74, 78, 79, 80, 82, 86, 87, 89
twins, 10
type 2 diabetes, 18

U

United, 31, 64, 87, 99
United States, 31, 64, 87, 99
urine, 34, 73

V

videos, 92
vision, 2, 9, 25, 52
vitamin D, 20
vitamins, 20, 21, 42, 67, 71
voicing, 68

W

walking, 18, 19

Washington, 24, 28, 32, 43, 44, 46, 56, 93, 95, 99
waste, 4
water, 74, 75
weakness, 71
wealth, 43
wear, 67
web, 32, 44, 59, 80, 92
websites, 36, 63, 77, 80, 82

weight loss, 70
well-being, 20, 30, 35, 91
wellness, 55
worry, 4, 7, 62, 90

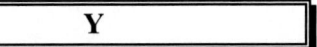

young people, 17